The Alzheimer's Rx:
Aerobic Exercise

The Alzheimer's Rx: Aerobic Exercise

Use the Approach AD S.A.F.E.ly™
Protocol to Engage Purposefully

Fang Yu, PhD, RN, FGSA, FAAN
Dereck L. Salisbury, PhD
Kaitlin E. Kelly, MSE, ATC

Cygnus Media, LLC
Publisher
Excelsior, Minnesota 55331

Dedication

This book is dedicated to people affected by Alzheimer's disease (AD) and their families who want to do everything they can to improve cognition, functional independence, and quality of life and refuse to let AD define who they are; the general public who are interested in learning about AD and using exercise to promote brain health and prevent AD; exercise providers who endeavor to make a difference in brain health and enrich the lives of people affected by AD; health care professionals, administrators, leaders, and policymakers who are in positions to influence exercise access and payment for people affected by AD. Thank you for joining our charge of making exercise widely available and a standard treatment for AD and the world dementia-friendly!

Table of Contents

Foreword

Dr. Fang Yu and her co-authors Dereck Salisbury and Kaitlin Kelly have written a very useful and comprehensive guide for patients, families, and health care professionals on how to establish an aerobic exercise program for individuals with mild cognitive impairment and for patients with Alzheimer's disease. Based on the research that Dr. Yu and her team have conducted for over fifteen years, the authors outline practical strategies for achieving safe and realistic exercise goals and provide evidence-based information on the effectiveness of aerobic exercise in improving cognition. Because Dr. Yu recognized the need to educate exercise providers on how to work specifically with people who have cognitive impairment, she also developed the FIT-AD™ Certificate Program, a very successful instructional program that is outlined in her book.

Dr. Yu is a leading scientist in the investigation of aerobic exercise for the prevention and treatment of Alzheimer's disease. She received her BS from Peking University Health Science Center and her MS and PhD from the University of Pennsylvania. After completing a Clair M. Fagin *Building Academic Geriatric Nursing Capacity* Post-Doctoral Fellowship sponsored by The John A.

Hartman Foundation, she joined the University of Minnesota School of Nursing (2006) where she is Professor and Chair of the Adult and Gerontological Health Cooperative and holds Long Term Care Professorship. In addition, Dr. Yu has published her work widely and her research is supported by grants from the National Institutes of Health. She is a Fellow in the Gerontological Society of the America and the American Academy of Nursing.

The Alzheimer's Rx: Aerobic Exercise contains a wealth of information not only on the benefits of an aerobic exercise program but also on the recognition, diagnosis, and treatment of Alzheimer's disease. It is highly recommended for anyone who wishes to explore this fascinating, non-pharmacological approach to the prevention and treatment of pre-Alzheimer's and Alzheimer's disease.

— Maurice Dysken, MD
Professor Emeritus, Department of Psychiatry
University of Minnesota
Former Director, Geriatric Research, Education, and Clinical
Center (GRECC) Program
Minneapolis VA Health Care System

Preface

This book was inspired by older adults with a clinical diagnosis of Alzheimer's dementia and their families, whom we have been privileged to work with in our 15+ years of aerobic exercise research. They have repeatedly told us what a difference our exercise program has made in their lives and how disappointed they are at the lack of access to exercise after completing our studies. Many said, "This [exercise] is the only good thing that has happened for having Alzheimer's."

By 2014, I had a revelation from the overwhelming, recurring themes of feedback that the answers to my research questions about if and how aerobic exercise alters Alzheimer's symptoms and course really did not matter that much to our participants and their family caregivers. Our participants had simply received the well-established health benefits from aerobic exercise such as improved physical function, emotional wellbeing, and quality of life, which had a rippling beneficial effect on family caregivers. So, is it warranted to continue to wait before recommending aerobic exercise as a treatment for Alzheimer's disease (AD)? Even if aerobic exercise cannot arrest the AD course in the end, does it mean that exercise should be withheld from people affected by AD? These questions planted the first seed that I have to do something to increase exercise access to this population.

In 2016, we made our first move in increasing exercise access by developing the FIT-AD™ Certificate Program. This Program was grounded in our belief that supervised exercise is critical for ensuring exercise safety, engagement, and enjoyment for people with Alzheimer's dementia due to their varying Alzheimer's symptoms, coexisting medical conditions, and impaired communication and judgment. The FIT-AD™ Certificate Program educates exercise providers (e.g., personal trainers, aerobics instructors, and health care professionals) on safely engaging older adults with Alzheimer's dementia in person-centered aerobic exercise over time. Our ultimate goal is to make aerobic exercise widely accessible and a standard treatment for AD.

Shortly after the FIT-AD™ Certificate Program, we set out to write this book to go more in-depth and target a broader audience than the FIT-AD™ Certificate Program. This book has 11 chapters. Chapters 1–3 synthesize AD clinical course, risk and protective factors, and abnormal brain changes. Chapters 4–5 introduce the exercise types, health benefits, and effects on AD. Chapters 7–8 explain the Approach AD S.A.F.E.ly™ protocol to start and adjust the aerobic exercise to the target dose safely. Chapters 9–11 discuss strategies to maximize exercise participation in response to AD symptoms as AD progresses over time. Each chapter begins and ends with scenarios based on true stories from our own lives and our research participants. The stories have been modified to protect our participants' privacy and confidentiality. The opening scenarios introduce a chapter's focus and are analyzed at the end to further stimulate critical thinking.

This book introduces the Approach AD S.A.F.E.ly™, our recently named brand. While the brand is new, its contents have been developed, tested, and refined over our exercise studies since 2004. The acronym "S.A.F.E." stands for 1) Screen your conditions, 2) Assess exercise readiness, 3) Follow medical evaluation, if needed, and 4) Evaluate fall risk and aerobic fitness. The Approach AD S.A.F.E.ly™ protocol originated from our pre-exercise health screening process and was built on the foundations of person-centered care and exercise safety. It includes individualized exercise prescription, exercise session flow, exercise response monitoring during an exercise session, AD symptom management, effective communication, working with family caregivers and health care professionals, motivating people affected by AD to exercise.

This book focuses solely on aerobic exercise, not only because the scientific evidence for it is the strongest, but also because aerobic exercise lays the foundation for the optimal effect of other interventions. Many changes induced by aerobic exercise at the molecular, cellular, structural, and functional levels prime the brain and body for optimizing the benefits from other interventions such as a healthy diet, cognitive activities, and social activities. The methods and tools covered by the Approach AD S.A.F.E.ly™ protocol apply to other types of exercises as well.

Currently, scientists and clinicians do not agree about the strength of evidence for recommending aerobic exercise for AD prevention and treatment. We hope the evidence presented in this book will allow you to draw your own conclusions. Should you find favor in the value and importance of aerobic exercise in AD, we hope this book equips you with the knowledge and tools to engage yourself or others in aerobic exercise to increase brain health, prevent AD, and improve quality of life for people affected by AD.

— Fang Yu

Acknowledgments

We want to thank our research participants and their families whose motivation, encouragement, support, dedication, and gratitude to our studies have inspired us. You have made such a difference in our lives and taught us that no diseases, not even Alzheimer's disease (AD), can define a person and a person's legacy. We deeply appreciate the families who went above and beyond to make sure their loved ones affected by AD are getting the most out of their lives.

We are indebted to our community partners: the YMCA in Twin Cities, particularly Southdale YMCA and Cora McCovey YMCA, Lyngblomsten, the Alzheimer's Association Minnesota and North Dakota Chapter, HealthPartners®, Ebenezer Senior Living, Dementia-Friendly Communities, adult day centers, Metropolitan Area Agency on Aging, Minnesota Good Age, and others. Thank you for believing in the value of exercise in AD, letting us use your facility and equipment to conduct exercise sessions, promoting our research in your communities, connecting potential participants to our studies, and supporting our participants and staff.

We cannot thank enough our research sponsors who made our exercise studies possible: the Alzheimer's Association, American Nurses Foundation, BrightFocus® Foundation, John A. Hartford Foundation, Minnesota Board on Aging, National Institutes of Health National Institute on Aging, Sigma Theta Tau International, University of Minnesota, and so on. Without your generous financial supports, none of our studies could have happened.

Our research studies would not have been successful without the outstanding and committed mentors, co-investigators, staff, students, and volunteers. Thank you for contributing your talents and passion to nurture us as scientists, help us design and implement the studies, and embody person-centered care to its core. Our staff and students have been the backbones of our studies. As many participants and families have testified, *"Dr. Yu has the best staff."*

We are deeply grateful for the strong support from the University of Minnesota School of Nursing. Its leadership, people, infrastructure, and commitment to research excellence have provided the ideal environment for helping us grow as scientists, clinicians, and educators. We also thank the outstanding resources at the University of Minnesota and its "Driven to Discover®" culture, which has greatly benefited our studies, including but not limited to the Clinical and Translational Science Institute, the Center for Magnetic Resonance Research, and M Health.

Last but not least, we thank our wonderful families who have unyieldingly supported every step we made. We are simply out of words to say how deeply appreciative we are about your being on our sides all the times and never complained about the long hours we spent at work and the never materialized vacations. Thank you for walking side by side with us in the fight to end AD.

Chapter 1

What Is Alzheimer's Disease?

One day, my husband, who was in his late 40s, decided that I needed a new computer to work at home, so he bought a fast, large-screen computer. We were very excited to see what this computer could do to make my life better, but months later, it still sat on my desk, collecting dust. Guess what happened? My husband could not find the wireless installation software anywhere. He had bought two copies of the software and recalled how he had stored them in a CD sleeve for easy access. The reason he had two copies was that he could not locate the first copy when he needed it before. This forgetfulness had been happening on and off. My husband eventually found the software, so we did not have to buy another copy.

Alzheimer's Disease

My mom has lived with us for 12 years. She plans and makes dinners on weekdays. One day when we came home, Mom had made three yummy dishes. When I opened the rice cooker—oops— the rice was not cooked! I calmly replaced the lid and asked Mom if she had cooked rice. Guess how surprised she was! She said that she remembered pressing the start button (the rice cooker was working normally). We all laughed. Similar things have happened since then. My mom loves to read the news and share what she read. However, she cannot recall some details of the news, like where and when something happened. She was in her mid-70s when this started.

At a community picnic, I met an acquaintance whom I had not seen for a few months. She said she knew me but could not recall my name or where we first met. I had to re-introduce myself several times during our conversation. After I reminded her what I do for a living, she told me how frustrated she was with her garage door. She would leave the house and wonder if she had closed the garage door. Quite often, it bothered her so much that she returned to check. As you may guess, the door was closed at times but open at others. She put a sticky note on her dashboard that read "close garage door" but forgot to look at it. She also tried to set a phone alarm. It worked well when she remembered to set it, but she did not always remember. Eventually, she installed an automatic garage door closer. She was in her late 60s.

A friend called me for advice about his dad, who was in his early 80s and lived alone. Over Thanksgiving, his sister visited from out of town and stayed with their dad. His sister said that their dad's personality seemed to have changed. He used to be very organized, but his house was a mess. She saw some late bills and asked if he had paid them. He got angry and said that, due to people like her rummaging through his belongings, he could not find things when he needed them. After his sister left, he became worried because his dad did not remember her visit. After being reminded, his dad seemed to remember but could not recall any details about it. When I asked my friend about what he had observed in the past few years, he recalled that his dad had locked himself out of the house a few times. "Dad is getting old. This is normal for his age, right?" he asked.

Have you or someone you know had some similar issues? Have you ever wondered whether memory loss and personality changes are just signs of old age or if they signal something bad? If so, you are not alone. Cognition is one of the most valued characteristics of humans. Because cognitive abilities make each person unique, there is often a reluctance to recognize cognitive decline even when it has become apparent.

In this chapter, you will learn about cognition, age-related cognitive changes, and abnormal decline due to Alzheimer's disease (AD). Although there are many causes of cognitive decline, this book focuses solely on AD as the cause. You will become familiar with the AD continuum and its three phases, symptoms, clinical diagnoses, and the three stages of Alzheimer's dementia (or AD dementia).

What Is Cognition?

Cognition refers to the mental processes of knowing and can be divided into different domains. AD has traditionally been diagnosed based on impairment in four discrete domains: memory, executive function, visuospatial function, and language, so our chapter is based on this tradition.

You may wonder how cognition differs from another commonly known word—intelligence. Intelligence describes the patterns of cognitive change over time and includes crystallized and fluid intelligence. Crystallized intelligence is the skill, ability, and knowledge that are overlearned and well-practiced due to the accumulation of information from experience. Fluid intelligence refers to the innate ability to reason, solve problems, and manipulate the environment. Memory (except for semantic memory), executive function, visuospatial function, and language (except vocabulary) are often considered fluid intelligence, while semantic memory and vocabulary crystallized intelligence. Now let us review each cognitive domain.

Memory

Memory refers to the ability to encode, store, and retrieve information. It is not a unitary construct and can be crudely divided into short-term and long-term memory (Figure 1.1). Short-term memory has very limited capacity, holding about only seven items for a few dozen seconds. When a conscious effort is not made to retain short-term memory, it disappears quickly and forever.

Long-term memory is activated when a conscious effort is made to remember something such as thinking about them repeatedly, giving them meaning, linking them with previous knowledge, and being interested in the subject. Long-term memory stores significant events, meanings of words, and learned physical skills and has unlimited capacity for content and duration.

Long-term memory is categorized into explicit and implicit memory. Explicit memory, also called declarative memory, involves the conscious recollection of facts, events, and experiences. There are two types of explicit memory which can be described in words: episodic memory and semantic memory (Figure 1.1). Episodic memory is the conscious recollection of experienced events at certain times and places as well as their social and physical contexts, e.g., a wedding, a trip to Europe, and a conversation with a friend a couple of days ago. Semantic memory, often called crystallized intelligence, stores factual and accumulated knowledge of the world, regardless of the context, e.g., historical events, names of cities, and definitions of words.

Implicit or nondeclarative memory can be recalled automatically without a conscious effort and be expressed by means other than words. For example, you can ride a bike without consciously recalling where and how you had learned to do it. Of the different types of implicit memory, procedural implicit memory, is best known and enables the learning of motor skills and gradually improving them.

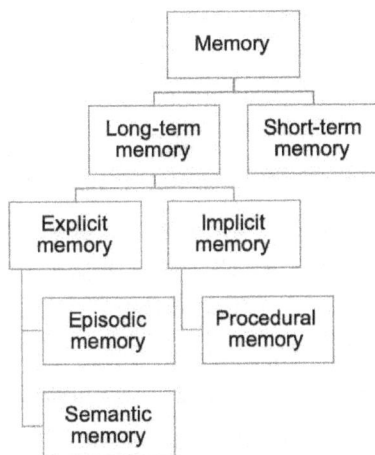

Figure 1.1. Multiple Memory Systems

Executive Function

Executive function is a higher-order cognitive construct and involves a set of skills that organize and regulate goal-directed behaviors and effective use of large amounts of information. In other words, it helps you to get things done.

Executive function operates through three components, including working memory, cognitive flexibility, and inhibitory control. "Hold on," you might ask, "is working memory a memory?" You are correct. However, working memory happens in the central executive part of the prefrontal cortex where executive function resides. This is the reason why working memory is also considered a component of executive function and why executive function plays a fundamental role in memory.

Working memory has been used interchangeably with short-term memory, but they are not the same. Short-term memory is just a part of working memory and maintains information (e.g., hold a phone number in mind before you write it down on paper). Working memory temporarily stores short-term memory and calls up information from other areas of the brain to integrate all information together and with past experience. Cognitive flexibility is the ability to adapt to a change by getting integrated information ready to make the next move. Mental or cognitive shifting, a component of cognitive flexibility, makes the move and switches back and forth between moves to adapt to new, changing, or unexpected events. Inhibitory control comes into play by suppressing the information and behaviors that are not pertinent to the task at hand.

Other executive function skills include attention, judgment, problem-solving, abstraction, and processing speed. Attention defines the ability to focus (sustained attention) and selectively concentrate on some aspects of the environment while ignoring others (selective attention). The ability to focus on multiple tasks simultaneously is called divided attention. Judgment and problem-solving refer to the ability to make decisions, come to sensible conclusions, and solve problems. Abstraction allows the classification of higher concepts based on the general attribute of concrete concepts. Processing speed refers to the speed of performing cognitive activities and motor responses.

Visuospatial Function

Visuospatial function is the ability to perceive, comprehend, and interpret visual and spatial information in different dimensions. It ensures accurate and efficient recognition of objects and faces, safe navigation of the environment, and coordination of visuomotor movements. Visuospatial construction skills include assembling a coherent whole out of individual parts, perceiving and reproducing three-dimensional figures, recognizing embedded objects, and identifying incomplete figures.

Language

Language defines the ability to produce spontaneous speech, comprehend and repeat language, name objects, read, and write. Verbal fluency is the ability to retrieve information from memory. For example, verbal fluency can be tested by asking people to form and express words according to pre-specified criteria such as telling as many words as possible that start with the letter "F" within one minute. Naming is the ability to see an object and name it and its parts. Reading indicates the ability to read and comprehend what is read. Writing refers to the ability to write complete sentences that are grammatically correct.

Where Does Cognition Come From?

The human brain weighs about three pounds and has three main parts: the cerebrum, cerebellum, and brainstem. The cerebrum is composed of two halves, the left and right hemispheres that are connected by a bundle of fibers. The surface of the cerebrum is called the cortex which is composed of the gray matter. The gray matter is the neural tissue that contains nerve-cell bodies and fibers, is about ½ cm thick, and gives the cortex a pinkish-gray coloring. Beneath the gray matter, the white matter gives the cerebrum a whitish coloring and contains fiber tracts connecting different parts of the brain to transmit messages. The cerebral cortex has about 10–20 billion neurons that carry out higher functions such as cognition, emotions, learning, and fine motor movements.

Within each hemisphere, the cortex is divided into four sections called "lobes" by the distinct hills called gyri and valleys named sulci: the frontal, parietal, temporal, and occipital lobes. Each lobe performs a specific function.

The frontal lobes are located in the front of the brain behind the forehead and are associated with executive function, personality, emotions, parts of speech (speaking and writing), body movement, intelligence, concentration, and self-awareness.

The parietal lobes make up the top middle section of the brain above the ears and affect speech (language interpretation and words), spatial and visual perceptions, and interpretation of visual and auditory signals as well as senses of touch, pain, and temperature.

The temporal lobes compose the bottom section of the brain around the ears and control memory, understanding of language, hearing, sequencing, and organization. The hippocampi are located within the temporal lobes and are where memory is formed.

The occipital lobes are situated in the back of the head and regulate the visual processing of color, light, and movement.

Although each lobe is responsible for performing a specific cognitive function, the lobes do not operate in silos. Instead, the lobes and areas of the brain are connected in a very complex manner through the subcortical circuitry. Subcortical means below the cortex.

What Changes Are Expected with Aging?

Much of what is known about age-related cognitive changes is based on laboratory research which shows older adults performing inferior to young adults on several cognitive domains. However, such age-related declines are rarely found to have consequences on real-life functioning such as job performance and achievements.

Memory

Aging affects various aspects of memory differently instead of leading to a global decline. Short-term memory is less affected by age than working memory. Long-term memory tends to become less reliable but remains robust and well preserved, allowing the recall of events and experiences of long ago.

Episodic memory declines with age in general, with its effortful aspects more affected than familiarity-based or automatic aspects. It takes longer to learn new information (longer encoding process) and recall newly and/or well-learned information (longer retrieval process), particularly when effortful processes are required. In contrast, semantic memory continues to improve until late life as knowledge accrues over the life span. Implicit memory remains relatively stable with aging in comparison to explicit memory.

Mild forgetfulness can be a normal part of aging. For instance, it can take longer to learn new things. You may lose things, not remember information as well as you used to, miss an occasional appointment, forget names but remember them later or with cues, and sometimes struggle to find the right word. Despite these changes, older adults are fully able to learn new things and create new memories.

Executive Function

Executive function is believed to be particularly vulnerable to the aging process and does not decline linearly across the life span. There is a sharp decline in executive function after age 60, with the decline accelerating after age 70.

Age-related decline in executive function is not uniform across all cognitive skills. Declines are often found in working memory, inhibition, mental shifting, planning, and reasoning with unfamiliar materials. Reasoning with familiar materials remains stable.

Age-related decline in working memory has real-life implications because working memory actively manipulates and processes information. As a result, older adults may have difficulty in following long and complex instructions, answering multiple-choice questions, and remembering and calculating prices when shopping. Age-related decline in working memory may be related to decreased attention control and inhibition.

Sustained attention is relatively unaffected by aging. Since aging changes inhibitory control, selective attention is age-sensitive, so distractibility increases in older adults. They also have difficulty in divided attention, which negatively affects their abilities to concurrently attend to and process information from dual or multiple sources or perform tasks requiring complex attention.

Processing speed begins to decline in the third decade of life and continues to decrease afterward. Many aspects of cognitive decline associated with aging may be at least partially due to decreased processing speed.

Visuospatial Function

Many aspects of visuospatial function remain intact with aging, such as object perception and recognition and spatial perception of the locations of objects alone or in relation to others in the physical environment. Other aspects of visuospatial function decline with age, particularly those depending on executive function such as visuospatial attention, visuospatial construction, and visuospatial processing. Visuospatial memory, visuospatial orientation, mental rotation, and complex figure copy also show a decline with age.

Language

In general, aging does not affect language. Vocabulary remains stable and even improves over time. Three areas of language show some evidence of mild age-related decline. Naming remains stable until age 70 and then declines. Verbal fluency declines with age. Another age-related change is the "tip-of-the-tongue" experience where older adults experience word-finding problems although they know the word. All three language changes are thought to arise from retrieval difficulty due to changes in sensory processes, executive function, or memory instead of a loss of semantic information.

Although age-related changes described in this section seem clearly defined, they are not. There are substantial variations in age-related changes among individuals. Many factors other than age are at operation for affecting cognitive aging, including educational attainment, intelligence, sensory abilities (vision and hearing), socioeconomic status, practice associated with any prior test experience, and so on. Age effects on cognition are also not uniform across cognitive domains for a given individual. As a result, there are considerable between- and within-person variability in cognitive aging in older adults.

Why Does Cognition Change with Age?

Biologically, cognitive aging is due to brain aging. Different parts of the brain shrink at different rates, some more than others. Decreased brain, gray matter, and white matter volumes are probably caused by neuronal death, decreased neuronal size, and fewer connections among them in any given area. Neurons regenerate only infrequently, and existing neurons become smaller due to decreases in the number, length, and complexity of the dendrites that help them communicate. Figure 1.2 illustrates the structure of neuron and synapse. Both neuronal death and structural changes likely lead to fewer connections among neurons.

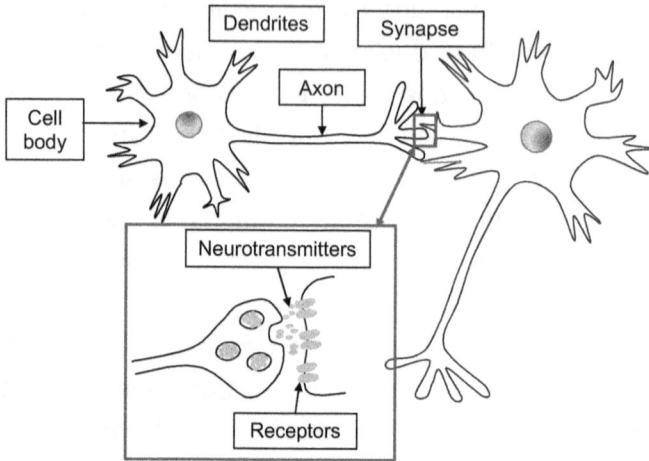

Figure 1.2. Structure of Neuron and Synapse

Brain volume decreases by about 0.5% per year with aging and reduction in the gray matter volume starts after 20 years of age. The rate of declines in brain and gray matter volumes are faster in the frontal lobes than the other lobes. Cortical thickness, a measure of how thick the gray matter is, normally ranges from 1 to 4.5 millimeters with an average of 2.5 millimeters, depending on the brain regions. A decline in cortical thickness becomes apparent by middle age with the frontal and parietal lobes showing greater rates of decline than the temporal and occipital lobes. The white matter volume continues to increase until the fifth decade of life and starts to decline afterward. Cerebral blood flow, metabolic rate, and vascular reactivity of blood vessels also decrease with aging.

What Cognitive Changes Are Caused by AD?

"Alzheimer's disease" was named after Alois Alzheimer, MD, who first described amyloid plaques and neurofibrillary tangles in the brain, the hallmark signs of AD, in 1907. Amyloid plaques form outside the neurons to destroy the healthy environment in which neurons live, and neurofibrillary tangles appear inside the neurons, crumpling them from within (see Figure 1.1). Compared with the roughly 0.5% loss per year in aging, the annual loss of brain mass is about five times higher in AD, resulting in about 200 to 400 g of brain mass loss over seven to 10 years. The hippocampus, the part of the brain where memory is made, shrinks by as much as 10% per year.

Before 2011, the terms "Alzheimer's disease" or "AD" had been used to designate both a clinical syndrome and abnormal AD brain changes, assuming the two correlates closely. A syndrome is a group of symptoms that occur together consistently. If a person has symptoms of the clinical syndrome of AD, then the underlying AD brain changes must exist, and vice versa. The extent of AD brain changes is consistent with the severity of clinical symptoms.

However, these assumptions have been increasingly challenged in the past three decades. About 10% to 30% of people with extensive AD brain changes never experienced obvious cognitive decline. Another 10% to 30% of people with few AD brain changes met the clinical diagnostic criteria for AD. These findings, along with other evidence, led to two updated guidelines: one for AD clinical diagnosis in 2011 and one for research purpose in 2018 from the National Institute on Aging-Alzheimer's Association workgroups. AD is reserved for referring solely to AD abnormal changes in the brain as a biological entity. The clinical course of AD is classified into three phases as the asymptomatic, preclinical phase (preclinical AD), the mild cognitive impairment (MCI) due to AD phase, and the Alzheimer's dementia (or AD dementia) phase. What used to be called AD clinically now refers to Alzheimer's dementia. Figure 1.3. depicts the AD continuum.

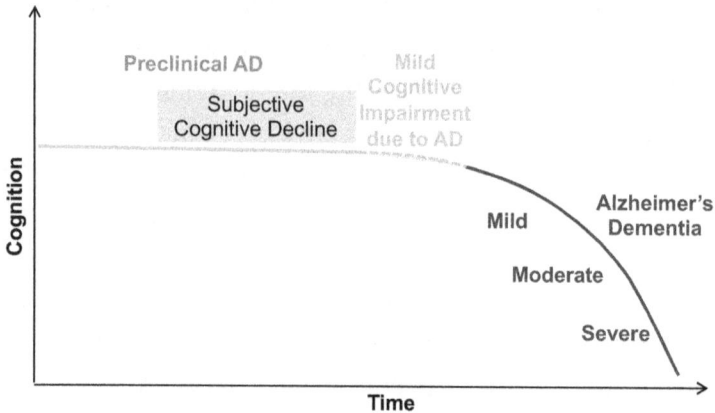

Figure 1.3. AD Continuum (AD: Alzheimer's Disease)

What Is Preclinical AD?

Preclinical AD, which is not a clinical diagnosis, refers to the years or decades in which AD brain changes begin to develop and build up. During this time, cognitive symptoms may not be present at all, may not be obvious if present, or may be noticeable only to the person affected. When cognitive symptoms are noticeable to the person affected, it is designated as subjective cognitive decline for research purposes. The rate of decline in preclinical AD is slow and begins to accelerate several years before transitioning to the MCI due to AD phase. On cognitive testing or neuropsychological evaluation, people with preclinical AD have normal results. Hence, regular cognitive testing over time may better detect cognitive decline than a one-time cognitive assessment.

Preclinical AD is not a clinical diagnosis for several reasons. First, many people with preclinical AD may never develop MCI or Alzheimer's dementia in their lifetimes although they are at risk for cognitive decline. Second, it remains unknown what extent of AD brain changes are needed to trigger the transition from preclinical AD to MCI due to AD because many other factors other than AD could affect the course of cognitive decline. Last, the linkages between specific AD biomarkers and subsequent cognitive impairment have not been fully established. A biomarker refers to an indicator of normal biological processes, pathogenic processes, or responses to treatments. Once research resolves these issues, preclinical AD may become useful for predicting the likelihood of occurrence of MCI due to AD and Alzheimer's dementia.

What Is MCI due to AD?

MCI due to AD is the period between preclinical AD and the full development of Alzheimer's dementia. It is a clinical diagnosis.

Clinical Diagnosis

There are five criteria that have to be met for a diagnosis of MCI due to AD to be made:

(1) The person, a family member, friend, or health care provider voices a concern. The concern may be signs or symptoms of cognitive decline:

- Memory decline such as having trouble learning and remembering new information or recent events.
- Executive dysfunction such as poor judgment or impaired ability to reason, solve problems, or handle complex tasks.
- Visuospatial dysfunction such as having difficulty finding ways, dressing properly, or finding objects in the plain view.
- Language impairment such as problems naming objects, self-expression, comprehension, reading, or writing.

(2) Cognitive tests show lower-than-expected performance in at least one cognitive domain. If an individual has been regularly tested to establish a trend, a decline in cognitive performance becomes evident over time.

(3) The cognitive decline is mild enough to have no significant effect on the person's ability to perform complex activities of daily

living. People with MCI due to AD may take more time, make more errors, or be less efficient than others, but they generally maintain their independence in daily function with minimal assistance. Basic activities of daily living such as eating, bathing, and toileting should be unaffected.

(4) Other possible causes for the cognitive decline are ruled out, such as depression, cerebrovascular conditions, traumatic brain injury, medications, and substance abuse.

(5) The diagnostic criteria for Alzheimer's dementia are not met. These criteria are described later in this chapter.

The key difference between preclinical AD and MCI due to AD is whether there is objective evidence of cognitive decline from cognitive tests. People with preclinical AD have normal test scores, but people with MCI due to AD score below the normal range.

Types

Depending on the cognitive domain involved, MCI due to AD can be classified into one of two types:

- Amnestic MCI, when cognitive impairment mostly affects episodic memory. A decline in episodic memory is the most common symptom among people with MCI who subsequently progress to Alzheimer's dementia.
- Non-amnestic MCI, when executive dysfunction, visuospatial dysfunction, or impaired language is the impaired domain.

Course

In MCI due to AD, the cognitive symptom can move in one of three directions: Revert back to normal, Stay in MCI, or Convert to Alzheimer's dementia. Predicting which direction a person's cognition will go is not a precise science because the course of MCI is influenced by a number of risk and protective factors, such as age, educational level, genetics, lifestyle, medical conditions, and environment (see Chapter 3 for details).

The chances of moving to one of the three directions vary from study to study, depending on the criteria for MCI due to AD, characteristics of the research participants, and duration of the follow-up. In general, about 15% to 20% of people with MCI due to AD are cognitively normal in a year, 60% to 70% stay in MCI, and another 5% to15% meet the diagnostic criteria for Alzheimer's dementia. Some studies have reported that the five-year conversion rate from MCI to Alzheimer's dementia ranged from 50% to 100%, and about 80% of people with amnestic MCI progressed to Alzheimer's dementia within seven years. For people with MCI who are destined to convert to Alzheimer's dementia, it takes, on average, six years for the conversion to happen, although it could take as few as four or as many as 10 years.

What Is Alzheimer's Dementia?

"Wait, is Alzheimer's dementia the same as dementia?" you might wonder. Not exactly. Dementia is an umbrella term with many different types or causes. Alzheimer's dementia is the most common type of dementia, accounting for about 60% to 80% of all dementias. Other types include vascular dementia (15%–20%), Lewy body dementia (5%), frontotemporal dementia (3%), Parkinson's disease, Huntington's disease, Creutzfeldt-Jakob disease and other prion disease, and dementia due to HIV/AIDS, infection, alcoholism, drugs, and systemic diseases such as thyroid disease and vitamin B12 deficiency. The percentages for different types of dementias do vary among studies, depending on the population and country studied. For a diagnosis of Alzheimer's dementia to be made, the diagnostic criteria for dementia must be met first.

Diagnosis of Dementia

Regardless of the cause, dementia is diagnosed with the same set of criteria:

(1) There must be impairment in at least two of the four cognitive domains, as shown by subjective reports from the affected person and/or someone who knows the person well. Common symptoms include:

- Impaired memory (trouble learning and remembering new information and recent events), as shown by asking repetitive questions, making the same statements repeatedly, forgetting appointments or events, getting lost in familiar places, and misplacing personal belongings.
- Executive dysfunction (impaired judgment, reasoning, and ability to handle complex tasks), as shown by poor understanding of safety risks, inability to manage finances and plan complex events or sequential activities, or poor decision-making.
- Impaired visuospatial function (impaired ability to make sense of visual and spatial stimuli), as shown by an inability to recognize common objects or faces, find objects in plain view despite having good eyesight, use common objects, or dress correctly.
- Impaired language (impaired ability to name objects, speak, read, write, and understand language), as shown by difficulty with finding common words when talking or presenting, hesitations in conversation, and frequent errors in speech, writing, and spelling.

These symptoms are backed by objective evidence of cognitive impairment from cognitive tests. On cognitive tests, people with Alzheimer's dementia score substantially lower than the population norm.

(2) The cognitive impairment must interfere with daily function, causing a decline from a previously higher level of functioning. Functional decline typically occurs in a hierarchical order over time, from impaired advanced activities of daily living to impaired instrumental activities of daily living to impaired basic activities of daily living. For example, people with Alzheimer's dementia initially experience decreased work performance, socialization, community involvement, and pursuit of hobbies and other interests. Then they have trouble with shopping, cleaning, cooking, or driving. Managing time and finances becomes increasingly difficult. Over time, they have difficulty performing basic activities of daily living such as eating, dressing, bathing, or toileting. In other words, daily functions that rely heavily on cognition deteriorate first. While the hierarchical order of functional decline is easy to understand, there are considerable variations among individuals. Functional declines in advanced, instrumental, and basic activities of daily living do overlap. For instance, a person may exhibit impairment in both instrument and basic activities of daily living.

(3) Cognitive impairment cannot be explained by delirium or other major psychiatric disorders. Delirium is an acute condition featuring confused thinking and reduced awareness of the environment. An example of a psychiatric condition that could present similar symptoms to dementia is depression.

Personality changes and behavioral and psychological symptoms of dementia are common in people with dementia, including depression, anxiety, psychosis (hallucinations and delusions), apathy, disinhibitions, sleep disturbances, agitation, and aggression. These symptoms are nearly universal, with up to 98% of individuals experiencing at least one during the course of dementia. These symptoms often cluster, exacerbate diseases, increase the use of health care services, lead to premature nursing home placement and death, and cause significant distress for family caregivers.

Diagnosis of Alzheimer's Dementia

When the diagnostic criteria for dementia are met, then it is important to determine the cause. To further diagnose dementia as Alzheimer's dementia, another set of criteria must be met. Alzheimer's dementia can then be diagnosed as either probable or possible. The core diagnostic criteria for probable Alzheimer's dementia include all of the following:

- Initial and most prominent impairment in memory (unable to learn new information and recall recently learned information), visuospatial function (unable to recognize objects, faces, or more than one object at a time), language (difficulty in word-finding and reading), and executive function (impaired reasoning, judgment, and problem-solving). At least two cognitive domains are impaired.
- A clear-cut history of worsening cognition, according to the person affected or an observer.
- Cognitive impairment that occurs gradually over months or years rather than suddenly over hours or days.
- No evidence of cerebrovascular disease or other dementia.

Possible Alzheimer's dementia is reserved for people who meet all the above criteria for probable Alzheimer's dementia, except that they have:

- An atypical or uncommon course, such as sudden cognitive impairment or lack of a clear history of progressive cognitive decline; *or*
- Evidence of cerebrovascular disease or other dementia

The key difference between MCI due to AD and Alzheimer's dementia is the preservation of independence in daily function. People with MCI due to AD do not have much difficulty with advanced and instrumental activities of daily living although they may be slower or less efficient in performing these activities in comparison to their past performance. Their basic activities of daily living are intact. In contrast, people with Alzheimer's dementia experience a substantial decline in these activities from a previously higher level of functioning.

Stages of Alzheimer's Dementia

Alzheimer's dementia progresses through three stages: mild, moderate, and severe stages or early, middle, and late stages (Figure 1.3). In the mild stage, which typically lasts two to four years, the most common initial symptom is the inability to remember or learn new information, which occurs slowly and gradually worsens over time. People with mild Alzheimer's dementia often have problems finding the right words or names, misplace or lose things, struggle with planning and organizing, and forget new information such as the names of people they just met and materials they just read. They have difficulty with advanced and instrumental activities of daily living such as handling money and paying bills. They may repeat questions and take longer to complete normal daily tasks. They could get lost but may still be able to or need a little help to drive and participate in social activities. They may show personality changes as well as behavioral and psychological symptoms of dementia such as anxiety, depression, and apathy.

The moderate stage can be the longest of the three stages, lasting two to 10 years, with a faster decline and greater level of assistance needed than the mild stage. People with moderate Alzheimer's dementia are very forgetful about daily events and some aspects of their own experiences and have trouble recalling their addresses, phone numbers, and names and faces of people they knew well in the past. They may be unable to learn new things, carry out multistep tasks such as getting dressed, or cope with new situations. They may begin to have problems recognizing family and friends. They often cannot perform advanced or instrumental activities of daily living and need help with some basic activities of daily living as well, such as using the bathroom, showering, and dressing. Bowel and bladder incontinence can also occur. Common behavioral and psychological symptoms include psychosis, agitation, aggression, sleep disturbances, wandering, and getting lost.

The severe stage usually lasts about one to three years. People with severe Alzheimer's dementia have increased difficulty communicating. They do not recognize people—even loved ones— and lose awareness of recent experiences and their surroundings. They have physical difficulty walking, sitting, and swallowing. They may develop contractures due to the shortening and hardening of muscles, tendons, and other tissues, which leads to joint rigidity and deformity. Eventually, they become bedbound and need 24-hour help with daily activities and personal care. They are susceptible to infections such as pneumonia, a major cause of death in people with Alzheimer's dementia.

Life Expectancy in Alzheimer's Dementia

The average life expectancy for people with Alzheimer's dementia is eight to 10 years after symptom onset but can be as long as 20 years. There is a high likelihood that life expectancy is underestimated due to two main reasons. First, the earliest symptoms of Alzheimer's dementia were not detected. Mild Alzheimer's dementia was mistaken as MCI due to AD. Second, the care of people with Alzheimer's dementia might have been less robust, resulting in reduced survival.

Variable Alzheimer's Symptoms and Course

Despite the general patterns of cognitive, functional, behavioral, and psychological symptoms, Alzheimer's dementia varies widely in terms of age of onset, symptoms, course, and needs for care. Among health care providers, there is a well-known saying: "If you have seen one person with Alzheimer's dementia, you have only seen one person with Alzheimer's dementia."

AD Continuum

While the three phases of AD (preclinical AD, MCI due to AD, and Alzheimer's dementia) are critical for advancing Alzheimer's research and clinical care, there are no fixed events indicating the beginning and end of an AD phase. AD is a continuum of abnormal processes in the brain. It is often very challenging to pinpoint the transition from preclinical AD to MCI due to AD and from MCI due to AD to Alzheimer's dementia. Cognitive decline in AD is slow, gradual, and progressive over years or decades. A rapid cognitive decline that occurs over weeks or months more likely originates from non-AD causes. AD often coexists with other conditions that also cause cognitive impairment, making it difficult to determine whether AD is the primary cause.

Jane's Story

To further illustrate the AD continuum, let us look at an actual person, whom we will call Jane. When we first met Jane in 2007, she was 68 years old. She responded to our recruitment advertisement that called for people with Alzheimer's dementia to participate in an aerobic exercise study. Because both her parents had died of Alzheimer's dementia, Jane and her four siblings were all very worried. Jane's cognitive decline was very subtle and gradual, so neither she nor her spouse could pinpoint when her symptoms began. However, she did not have Alzheimer's dementia and was in the preclinical AD phase. More specifically, she had subjective cognitive decline at the time. Although Jane was not eligible to participate in our study, we did have a great conversation about things she could do to keep her brain healthy.

When we launched another exercise study for older adults with Alzheimer's dementia a couple of years later, Jane contacted us again. She had become increasingly disorganized and could not keep a schedule. She was either late or did not show up for her hobby as a book reader to kids at her church and eventually had to give it up. After she had paid bills late several times, her spouse took over their finances. Otherwise, Jane was very independent in her daily activities. Jane underwent clinical evaluation about nine months ago and scored below the population norm in executive function tests. As a result, her provider diagnosed her with MCI due to AD. Jane and her spouse were both disappointed that she again did not meet the eligibility criteria for enrollment in our study.

Fast forward to 2015, we were still recruiting participants for our FIT-AD™ Trial, which was started in summer 2013. Jane and her spouse contacted us again. When we met Jane this time, she had just been diagnosed with Alzheimer's dementia. Our assessment showed that she was in the moderate stage of Alzheimer's dementia. She met all the eligibility criteria and was enrolled in our exercise study. Jane loved our exercise program and attended 98% of the sessions. Her spouse was also close to our staff and stayed in touch afterward. By early 2019, Jane's condition got worse. She no longer recognized her spouse or children and was resistant and aggressive when they tried to help her dress, eat, or use the toilet. Jane had fallen a few times and was hospitalized due to fall-related injuries. After many discussions with Jane's health care providers, the family decided to place her in a memory care unit. A few months later, Jane got pneumonia and passed away.

Reflecting back, we could see that Jane had gone through the preclinical AD, MCI due to AD, and Alzheimer's dementia phases of AD. However, no one could recall when the preclinical AD phase ended and the MCI phase began. When we first met Jane, it seemed clear that she had subjective cognitive decline. When Jane became eligible for our study, she was already well into the moderate stage of Alzheimer's dementia. Luckily for Jane, her time in the early phases of AD was longer, and she spent fewer years in the moderate and severe stages of Alzheimer's dementia. Although we would like to attribute Jane's favorable disease course to our exercise intervention, we know that it was the result of all the proactive things Jane had done to stay mentally stimulated, socially engaged, and physically healthy.

Key Messages

- Clinically, cognition is often discussed in four discrete domains as memory, executive function, visuospatial function, and language. Memory encodes, stores, and retrieves information. Executive function helps to get things done. Visuospatial function recognizes objects and faces, navigate the environment, and have skilled visuomotor movements. Language refers to speech, naming reading, and writing.
- Age-related changes in memory include longer encoding and recall processes and less reliable but still robust and well-preserved long-term memory.
- Executive function starts to decline after age 60, and the decline accelerates after age 70, but reasoning with familiar materials remains stable.
- Aging does not affect language in general. Vocabulary can even increase with age.
- Many aspects of visuospatial function remain intact with aging, but visuospatial construction skills decline.
- Age-related cognitive changes are probably caused by the decreased brain mass and volume with aging, at about 0.5% a year, likely due to decreased neuron size, reduced synaptic density, and neuron death.

- AD is a continuum of abnormal changes in the brain and causes a gradual, progressive cognitive decline over time, from preclinical AD to MCI due to AD and, eventually, Alzheimer's dementia. Where one phase of AD ends and another begins is not clear-cut, which makes an early diagnosis of MCI due to AD and Alzheimer's dementia difficult.
- MCI due to AD is a fluid state in which individuals could revert back to normal cognition, stay in MCI, or convert to Alzheimer's dementia. MCI is diagnosed when both subjective and objective evidence of the cognitive decline are present, but cognitive decline does not affect functional independence and is not explained by other conditions.
- Dementia is an umbrella term with many different causes. Alzheimer's dementia is the most common and accounts for about 60% to 80% of all dementias. Alzheimer's dementia progresses through three stages: mild, moderate, and severe stages or early, middle, and late stages.
- To be diagnosed with probable Alzheimer's dementia, the diagnostic criteria for dementia must be met first. In addition, a core set of criteria must be met, including prominent impairment in two or more cognitive domains and clear-cut history of worsening cognition that occurs gradually and is not explained by other conditions.
- The presenting symptoms, disease course, and life expectancy among people with Alzheimer's dementia are highly variable across individuals.

The Beginning Scenarios

Now, let us return to the four scenarios at the beginning of this chapter. What do you make of my husband's being unable to find his CDs, my mom's forgetting to cook rice and recount the details of news, my acquaintance's garage door situation, and my friend's dad not remembering his daughter's visit, disorganization, and personality changes? If we assume that no other diseases or conditions could have explained the cognitive changes in these scenarios, how would you describe their cognitive status given the information available? Here is my assessment: My husband was experiencing age-related memory changes. My mom had subjective cognitive decline. My acquaintance most likely had MCI due to AD, and my friend's dad had symptoms of Alzheimer's dementia. So, as you can see, telling the different phases of AD apart is possible, but it can be tricky.

Chapter 2

What Causes Alzheimer's Disease?

A group of people met at the 2019 Alzheimer's Association International Conference. Some of them had been friends for years, while others had known each other's work only by reputation. Some were students attending the conference for the first time. Some had been doing benchwork with animal models of Alzheimer's disease (AD) in a laboratory. Others have been running human studies. After some initial meets and greets, these conversations took place:

"I went to a presentation yesterday in which an anti-amyloid [a protein implicated in AD] drug was introduced. What do you think? It looks very promising, right? After all these failed drug trials, finally, there is a hope of success ......"

"I do not know if this particular drug is the one, but I do think that an effective drug is on the horizon. So much progress has already been made, so now we have a pretty good idea about how amyloids are produced, how they cluster together to form plaques, and how to remove them from the brain. At a presentation this morning, I learned that a drug targeting the early stage of amyloid formation is showing positive results. They are getting approval from the FDA [U.S. Food and Drug Administration] to launch a large trial soon ......"

"Hopefully, these anti-amyloid drugs will have better fates than their predecessors. I am skeptical because I think we are really barking up the wrong tree. Although amyloid is an early event in AD brain changes, it does not predict cognitive impairment very well, which is why anti-amyloid drugs have not worked. Abnormal tau [another protein implicated in AD] is really the culprit. My lab has discovered a promising target for new drugs to reduce abnormal tau ......"

"Tau is definitely very important, but I do not think our confidence in amyloid is misplaced. The evidence is pretty strong that amyloid must be present for abnormal tau to occur, but you are right that tau coincides cognitive symptoms better than amyloid ......"

"I am very disappointed that so much emphasis is still being placed on amyloid and tau. Our work has consistently shown that mitochondrial dysfunction and oxidative stress occur earlier than either amyloid or tau ......"

"The presentation I went to this morning also suggested that neither amyloid nor tau causes AD. They are there to protect the brain from the real enemy: infection. They said that infection in early life predisposes people to AD in late life ......"

"Is it infection or inflammation? I think it is the latter. The field has grown so much on neuroinflammation and how it contributes to AD brain changes ......"

"Wait, but none of the existing AD drugs addresses any of these brain changes directly, right? Why are these drugs FDA-approved then? I feel like I am missing something very important here," a student chimed in. More students asked questions: "What about cardiovascular diseases?" "Insulin resistance and diabetes?" ......

To unravel the abnormal processes that cause a disease is essential to discover treatments that can affect, arrest, or cure the disease. Determining the cause of AD has been a long and tortuous path, as reflected by the snippets of conversations at the conference. Amyloid plaques and neurofibrillary tangles are popularly regarded as AD hallmarks (Figure 2.1). However, there are still controversies about whether and how they cause AD. In addition, a host of other non-hallmark brain changes happen in AD, including neurodegeneration, mitochondrial dysfunction and oxidative stress, insulin resistance and glucose hypometabolism, neuroinflammation, vascular dysfunction, neurochemical changes, and infection. Together, hallmark and non-hallmark changes form a

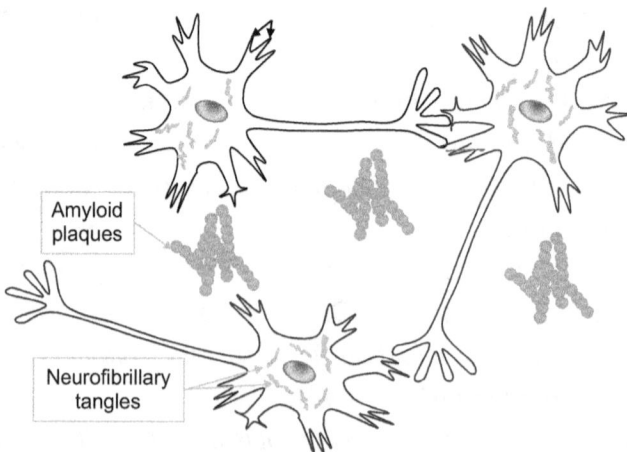

Amyloid plaques

Neurofibrillary tangles

Figure 2.1. Hallmarks of Alzheimer's Disease

downward spiral to accelerate the development and progression of AD.

In this chapter, you will be introduced to AD biomarkers for studying AD brain changes in living people. Biomarkers are objective indicators of normal biological processes, pathogenic processes, or responses to treatments. You will read a detailed description of AD hallmark and non-hallmark brain changes to gain a better understanding of AD. Please note that the non-hallmark brain changes are not unique to AD because they can be caused by non-AD diseases.

How Are AD Brain Changes Studied?

The disease processes of AD have mainly been investigated using AD-transgenic animal models, autopsies of human brains after death, and AD biomarkers in living people. The word "transgenic" means related to transgenes—genes that are taken from one organism and transferred into the genetic makeup of another. AD-transgenic animal models carry one or more known AD genes from humans. Many different AD-transgenic animal models have been bred.

Because the human brain is enclosed and protected by the skull and other structures, it cannot be easily accessed in living humans. This is the reason why AD can only be definitively diagnosed after death when an autopsy could be performed to confirm the presence of AD hallmark brain changes in the past.

During the past three decades, the emergence of AD biomarkers has enabled researchers to study AD brain changes in living people. The publication of the National Institute on Aging-Alzheimer's Association (NIA-AA) Research Framework for AD in the journal *Alzheimer's & Dementia* in 2018 was groundbreaking. It classifies

AD biomarkers into three categories under the AT(N) system: A (amyloid), T (tau), and N (neurodegeneration or neuronal injury).

As its title implies, the AT(N) system is a research framework at present and is not intended for aiding the diagnosis of AD clinically. However, AD biomarkers will likely make definitive AD diagnosis possible in living people in the near future. This research framework is fluid in essence to allow newer biomarkers to be added as more knowledge about AD brain changes is generated and accommodate the controversies over amyloid plaques and neurofibrillary tangles. It specifies the use of imaging and cerebrospinal fluid (CSF) biomarkers but does not yet include any blood biomarkers.

Imaging Biomarkers of AD

The brain can be imaged using both noninvasive and minimally invasive methods. Magnetic resonance imaging (MRI) is noninvasive and can identify structural (structural MRI) and functional changes (functional MRI) in the brain. The changes identified by the MRI, however, are not specific to AD and can be caused by other neurodegenerative conditions.

Positron emission tomography (PET) is minimally invasive because it requires the injection of a radioactive tracer to the peripheral blood that binds to amyloid (amyloid PET), tau (tau PET), or glucose (fluorodeoxyglucose or FDG PET) in the brain. Increased tracer retention allows the determination of amyloid load, accumulation of tau tangles, or reduced use of glucose in the brain. Currently, several amyloid tracers are available. Tau tracers have been developed, but they do not yet work as well as amyloid tracers due to relatively low and/or nonspecific brain uptake and binding.

The imaging biomarkers are the indirect measures of AD brain changes because they cannot detect brain changes at the molecular and cellular levels. Further research is needed to determine how to best score amyloid load and tauopathy and whether a summary score in a cerebral lobe or across different lobes is the most predictive of future cognitive decline, mild cognitive impairment due to AD, and Alzheimer's dementia.

Notably, some people cannot undergo imaging due to safety issues. We use both MRI and amyloid PET in our studies. When a participant screens positive for a foreign object in the body such as a shoulder replacement part, we have to identify its exact make and model to ensure that it can safely go through the scanner. This sometimes is impossible because the surgery might have taken place decades ago, or the medical records simply do not contain the relevant information. Imaging itself can be expensive. When the scanner, technician, and radiologist time for obtaining and reading the scans and the cost of the tracers are added together, a single PET scan can easily cost thousands of dollars.

CSF Biomarkers of AD

The brain and spinal cord make up the central nervous system and are separate from the rest of the body. They are enveloped by the protective membranes known as the meninges and encased within the skull and spinal column. Hollow cavities in the brain called the ventricles contain the CSF, a clear and colorless fluid. The CSF is mainly comprised of proteins and electrolytes, with few cells. Changes in the CSF contents can indicate changes in the brain.

The CSF biomarkers of AD are obtained through an invasive procedure called lumbar puncture or spinal tap. To do a spinal tap, a health care provider injects a local anesthetic at the site where a needle will be inserted between two vertebrae (lumbar bones) to remove some CSF. The spinal tap is generally safe but can cause post-spinal tap headache, back discomfort or pain, bleeding, and brainstem herniation.

Experts have been working hard to standardize the procedures for preanalytical CSF sample handling and CSF-biomarker analysis across different platforms and laboratories. These efforts allow the use of CSF biomarkers to predict cognitive decline and onset of mild cognitive impairment due to AD or Alzheimer's dementia and distinguish Alzheimer's dementia from other types of dementia.

Blood Biomarkers of AD

Health care providers widely use blood biomarkers to diagnose diseases and assess treatment responses. Blood collection is minimally invasive, familiar, and cost-effective. Blood biomarkers you might be familiar with include fasting blood glucose and hemoglobin A1c for diabetes, blood cholesterol for high cholesterol, and blood alcohol for alcohol intoxication.

Would not it be wonderful if blood biomarkers also existed for AD? There are several reasons why blood biomarker discovery has lagged behind the imaging and CSF biomarkers of AD. The brain is secluded from the circulating blood by the blood-brain barrier. The blood-brain barrier is a highly selective border that allows only certain molecules to travel in and out of the brain. As a result, the levels of AD biomarkers in the blood are substantially lower than their levels in the CSF. Some studies estimate that no more than 25% of amyloid in the brain enters the circulating blood through the blood-brain barrier. In addition, how the blood is collected, processed, and analyzed contributes to the variations in the results. Recently, neurofilament light chain has been found to transfer directly from the CSF to blood and reflects one type of AD brain change—neurodegeneration, making it a very promising biomarker.

Caution about AD Biomarkers

Despite their promises and importance, biomarkers are the proxies, or stand-ins, of AD brain changes. The human brain is such a complex organ that the biomarkers may reflect only parts of AD brain changes. How valuable the biomarkers are for predicting cognitive decline and AD clinical progression is a critical area of research. Current findings vary from study to study, influenced by many factors such as the risk profiles of the participants (e.g., age, genetic risk, education, and socioeconomic status).

AD biomarkers have not been compared with each other, used in combinations, or validated against AD brain changes after death. The cutoff scores on most biomarkers need further validation. Solutions for resolving conflicting results among biomarkers are lacking; for example, one biomarker is positive while another is negative or ambiguous, or a biomarker level does not neatly fall into a "positive" or "negative" category. Because of these unresolved issues, AD biomarkers are not ready for clinical use. Mild cognitive impairment and Alzheimer's dementia continue to be diagnosed based on the criteria described in Chapter 1.

How Do Amyloid Plaques Form?

The amyloid cascade hypothesis has dominated the investigation of AD brain changes for many years. It suggests that an imbalance between the production and removal of amyloid-beta (Aβ) peptides results in amyloid deposition, which is either the triggering event of AD or occurs very early in AD. A peptide consists of two or more amino acids linked in a chain and has a C terminus on one end or an N terminus at the other end. Amyloid peptides aggregate to form amyloid plaques outside the neurons, which is one of two AD hallmark brain changes. The amyloid build-up has also been called amyloid deposition, amyloid load, amyloidosis, amyloid aggregate, and amyloid accumulation.

People with Alzheimer's dementia have many more amyloid plaques than those found in normal aging. Amyloid plaques typically begin in the cortex, the outermost layer of the brain, and then spread down to the inner brain regions. An exception is the hippocampi where memory is formed. Hippocampi are located in the inner brain but are affected early in AD. Amyloid deposition is considered necessary for triggering the second AD hallmark brain change, tau hyperphosphorylation. Amyloid deposition occurs decades before cognitive symptoms appear, but is likely insufficient to cause cognitive impairment by itself.

Normal Amyloid Production in the Brain

Amyloid is normally produced in the brain from a transmembrane protein called amyloid precursor protein (APP). APP is widely distributed throughout the body and may play an important role in brain development, synaptic plasticity, and neuroprotection. It extends from the inside to the outside of a neuron across the neuron's membrane, with a small portion inside the neuron and a large portion extending outside the neuron and folding into a ball shape. APP is sequentially cut to shorter pieces by scissor-like enzymes known as secretases. Enzymes catalyze chemical and biological reactions.

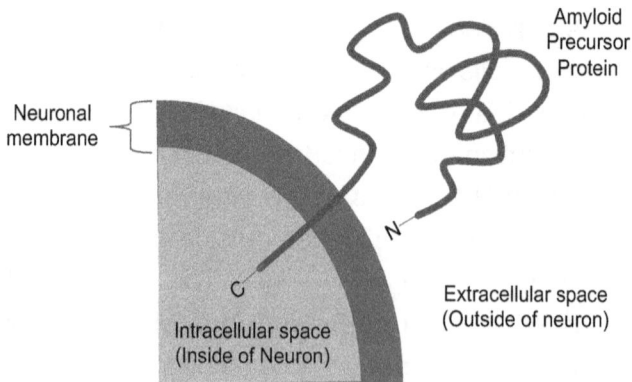

Figure 2.2. Amyloid Precursor Protein Across Neuronal Membrane

APP is first cut outside a neuron's membrane by α- or β-secretase to two pieces: a long N-terminal segment outside the neuron and a short C-terminal segment across the neuron's member and inside the neuron. The length of the C-terminal segment depends on the secretase involved: β-secretase produces a longer segment than α-secretase.

Next, the C-terminal segment is cut by γ-secretase within the neuron's membrane to release a short piece to the extracellular space (meaning outside the neurons). This short piece is made up of 22–27 amino acids when the APP is primarily cut by α- and γ-secretases under normal conditions. It is also not toxic to the brain cells.

Abnormal Amyloid in AD

In AD, APP is increasingly clipped by β- and γ-secretases instead of α- and γ-secretases because the activity of β-site APP cleaving enzyme 1 is elevated. β-site APP cleaving enzyme 1 is the active component of β-secretase. In addition, the action of γ-secretase becomes imprecise. The resulting short piece that is released to the extracellular space by β- and γ-secretases is longer than that produced by α- and γ-secretases. This short piece is called Aβ and consists of 38 to 43 amino acids. The 40 and 42 amino-acid-long segments are the predominant species and are often noted as $A\beta_{40}$ and $A\beta_{42}$. Once produced, $A\beta_{40}$ and $A\beta_{42}$ deposit diffusely in the brain and attract each other to form interlaced fibrils. Fibrils then stick to each other to form β sheets, which in turn fold into each other to form amyloid plaques.

$A\beta_{42}$ is more toxic to the neurons and has a greater propensity for aggregation than $A\beta_{40}$ because its two additional amino acids are hydrophobic or repel water. $A\beta_{42}$ is the major component of amyloid plaques and $A\beta_{40}$ is only found in a subset of amyloid plaques.

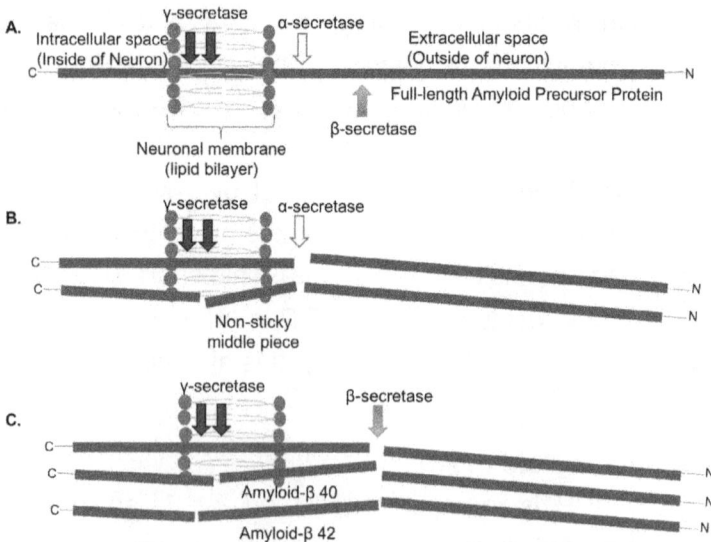

Figure 2.3. Production of Amyloid-β from Amyloid Precursor Protein
A. Different cutting points of the secretases on amyloid precursor protein.
B. Release of a non-sticky middle piece by α- and γ-secretases outside of a neuron.
C. Release of sticky amyloid-β 40 and 42 by β- and γ-secretases outside of a neuron.

It remains unclear why $A\beta_{42}$, the less abundant $A\beta$, is the major component of amyloid plaques. $A\beta_{40}$ alone does not seem to aggregate to form amyloid plaques when $A\beta_{42}$ is low or not available. The formation of mixed $A\beta_{40}$ and $A\beta_{42}$ aggregates is also slower than that of $A\beta_{42}$ only aggregates. Thus, $A\beta_{42}$ alone is stipulated to be responsible for amyloid plaques in AD.

Amyloid Biomarkers

Given the roles amyloid plays in AD, you can understand why the 2018 NIA-AA Research Framework for AD designated amyloid deposition on PET imaging, $A\beta_{42}$, and $A\beta_{42}/A\beta_{40}$ ratio in the CSF as amyloid biomarkers. However, these biomarkers are limited in that they measure only the accumulation and deposition of some forms of amyloid. Recent evidence suggests that soluble, oligomeric forms (short chains of amino acids) of $A\beta$ may be the major toxic agents to the neurons.

What Are Neurofibrillary Tangles?

The second hallmark brain change of AD is neurofibrillary tangles that cripple the neurons from within. Neurofibrillary tangles are initially localized to the brain areas where memory is formed and spread to other cortical areas, affecting executive function, visuospatial function, and language. The density of neurofibrillary tangles correlates strongly with the severity of cognitive impairment. Neurofibrillary tangles are abnormal protein clusters mainly composed of hyperphosphorylated tau.

Normal Tau

Tau is a major microtubule-associated protein (MAP), along with MAP 1 (A/B) and MAP2. Microtubules are the pipe-like structures inside neurons that transport nutrients and wastes and support the physical structure of neurons.

Tau, MAP1, and MAP2 perform similar functions of promoting the assembly and stability of the microtubules like the brackets to the walls. Their redundant functions constitute a naturally-built failsafe mode to maintain the microtubules. When there is a loss of normal tau due to injuries or diseases, the affected neurons synthesize more tau and step up the production of the other MAPs to compensate for the loss of tau. Tau's activity is regulated through phosphorylation (addition of phosphate). Normal tau contains 2–3 mol phosphate per mol of tau.

Tau Hyperphosphorylation in AD

In AD, tau becomes hyperphosphorylated (overloaded with extra phosphate), causing hyperphosphorylated tau to build up in the affected neurons. The level of hyperphosphorylated tau is four- to eight-fold higher in the brains of people affected by AD than of healthy people. Hyperphosphorylated tau disrupts microtubule's transportation function, compromises the flow of electrical and chemical signals, impedes normal neuronal function, causes synaptic loss, and eventually leads to cell death.

Hyperphosphorylated tau forms filament or threadlike structures, which stick together to develop neurofibrillary tangles. About 60% of hyperphosphorylated tau is found in neurofibrillary tangles. Hyperphosphorylated tau in the neurofibrillary tangles is inert, indicating that neurofibrillary tangles might be a neuron's self-defense response, at least initially. However, once the number and size of neurofibrillary tangles reach a certain threshold, they are toxic to the neurons.

The other 40% of hyperphosphorylated tau exist in the cytoplasm (jelly-like fluid within a cell). They harbor normal tau, MAP1, and MAP2, undermining the neuron's attempts at compensating for the loss of normal tau.

It is yet unknown what makes tau prone to hyperphosphorylation in the first place. One possibility is that tau might undergo changes in shape, which makes it an easy prey for phosphorylation and/or a less favorable target for dephosphorylation (to return it to normal tau). Another possibility is an imbalance between tau hyperphosphorylation and dephosphorylation. The enzymes, such as protein kinase A, glycogen synthase kinase-3, and cyclin-dependent protein kinase-5 that aid hyperphosphorylation, are increased in AD. In contrast, enzymes such as protein phosphatase-2A that facilitate dephosphorylation are impeded.

Abnormal Glycosylation of Tau in AD

Glycosylation refers to the attachment of a carbohydrate or sugar molecule to another molecule. Tau is normally glycosylated through O-GlcNAcylation (addition of sugar to amino acid serine and threonine). In AD, tau has significantly reduced O-GlcNAcylation, which seems to occur before tau hyperphosphorylation. Abnormal glycosylation seems to promote hyperphosphorylation and depresses dephosphorylation of tau, resulting in increased tau hyperphosphorylation. Hyperphosphorylation, in turn, triggers abnormal glycosylation, forming a downward spiral.

Tau Biomarkers

The 2018 NIA-AA Research Framework for AD designated neurofibrillary tangles detected on Tau PET and phosphorylated tau measured in the CSF as tau biomarkers. CSF total tau was not considered an AD biomarker because increased CSF total tau is not unique to AD; it can be caused by other brain conditions such as traumatic brain injury, cerebrovascular disease, and Creutzfeldt-Jakob disease. Phosphorylated tau, on the other hand, is very specific to AD and is not elevated in these other brain conditions.

To summarize, scientists currently believe that amyloid deposition is needed for tau hyperphosphorylation to occur. However, this relationship remains unclear. Causative events other than amyloid may exist but have not yet been discovered. Amyloid increases tau's hyperphosphorylation and tendency to build up by activating specific tau enzymes. Similarly, amyloid and abnormal tau can induce other abnormal brain changes. Tau hyperphosphorylation likely speeds up before objective evidence of cognitive impairment appears in the mild cognitive impairment phase of AD.

Controversies About AD Hallmark Changes?

Although amyloid plays a fundamental role in AD, it remains unknown whether it is the primary driver of AD. There is a well-known disconnect between amyloid load and cognitive impairment. About 10% to 30% of cognitively normal people were amyloid positive on autopsy (meeting the criteria for a pathologic AD diagnosis). It is unknown whether these people would have had cognitive impairment if they had lived longer. In contrast, another 10% to 30% of people who met the clinical diagnostic criteria for Alzheimer's dementia did not have a corresponding level of amyloid deposition in the brain on autopsy.

Several recent clinical trials of promising anti-amyloid drugs found little benefit on cognition despite reducing amyloid deposition. Amyloid-modifying drugs might have limited effect once neurodegeneration has already begun. As a result, drug trials have been underway targeting early-phase AD (mild cognitive impairment and preclinical AD) and hopefully will report favorable results in the near future.

The association between the number of neurofibrillary tangles and the severity of AD symptoms has also been inconsistent. Similar to amyloid plaques, neurofibrillary tangles may reflect cell autophagy and be a late indicator of tau's toxic impact. Autophagy means self-devour and is the natural mechanism for cells to disassemble dysfunctional components and preserve endangered neurons.

What Other Brain Changes Happen in AD?

Other abnormal brain changes in AD include neurodegeneration, mitochondria dysfunction and oxidative stress, insulin resistance and glucose hypometabolism, neuroinflammation, vascular dysfunction, neurochemical changes, and infection. These changes are not considered as AD hallmarks because a range of other brain injuries and conditions can also cause these changes. Hence, biomarkers for these non-hallmark brain changes are also not unique to AD. Let us review each of these abnormal brain changes.

Neurodegeneration

Neurodegeneration refers to synaptic dysfunction and loss as well as neuronal injury and death. A synapse refers to the point where nerve impulses pass from one neuron to another. Synaptic loss, often measured after death, correlates with cognitive decline in people who were cognitively normal and those who had AD.

Synaptic loss

Brain biopsies in people with Alzheimer's dementia show a roughly 25% to 30% decrease in synapses of the frontal and temporal cortices. Each neuron lost about 15% to 35% of its synapses in the two to four years following the onset of Alzheimer's dementia with the biggest loss in the hippocampi (up to 44%–55%). Synaptic loss happens in both dead and surviving neurons, decreasing the ratio of synapses to neurons by about 48%.

Synaptic changes might occur before amyloid accumulation can be detected. Scientists now think that synaptic dysfunction and neurodegeneration in the context of amyloid accumulation trigger cognitive decline. Synaptic loss seems to be most correlated with the occurrence of cognitive symptoms, followed by neurofibrillary tangles and then amyloid plaques.

Biomarkers of neurodegeneration

The 2018 NIA-AA Research Framework for AD designates fluorodeoxyglucose PET, structural MRI, and CSF total tau for measuring neurodegeneration biomarkers. Fluorodeoxyglucose PET can show an AD-specific pattern of decreased glucose use in certain parts of the brain (posterior cingulate, precuneus, and/or temporoparietal cortices). Structural MRI can indicate cortical thinning or gray matter atrophy mainly in the temporoparietal cortex and hippocampi. Elevated total tau in the CSF is a strong indicator of neuronal injury.

Mitochondrial Dysfunction & Oxidative Stress

In 2004, experts formally proposed the mitochondria cascade hypothesis, which states that mitochondria dysfunction occurs with aging and is influenced by a person's genetics and the environment.

Once mitochondrial dysfunction reaches a critical tipping point, AD hallmark brain changes, neurodegeneration, and oxidative stress ensue.

Oxidative stress, which refers to the physiological stress caused by the accumulative damage from free radicals that are not adequately removed by antioxidants, increases with normal aging but is much more extensive and occurs very early in AD. Oxidative stress arises when the production of free radicals overwhelms the ability of the antioxidant system to regulate or remove them due to the increased free radical production, decreased antioxidant defense, or both.

Free radicals

Free radicals contain one or more unpaired electrons in their outer shells and include reactive oxygen species and other molecules such as reactive nitrogen species. Free radicals can be the byproducts of mitochondrial activities during normal essential functions.

Mitochondria, the specialized structures within a cell, exist in large numbers in most cells, including brain cells. Their main task is to produce energy through respiration, which is why mitochondria are known as the "energy factory" of cells. Normally, about 98% of the oxygen molecules we breathe in move through the mitochondrial electron transport chain. The rest are reduced to superoxide radicals, which produce hydrogen peroxide when an electron is added.

When the production of superoxide radicals and hydrogen peroxide becomes excessive, highly reactive oxygen species and other free radical molecules are generated. Free radicals can also originate from external sources such as exposure to X-rays, ozone, cigarette smoking, air pollutants, and industrial chemicals.

Antioxidant systems

While mitochondria are the source of free radicals, they also keep the levels of free radicals stable through the antioxidant defense systems. These systems reduce the production and facilitate the removal of free radicals using both antioxidant enzymes such as superoxide dismutase, glutathione peroxidase, and catalase as well as non-enzymatic antioxidant factors such as vitamins E, C, and A and carotenoids. Because metals such as iron or copper are needed to produce free radicals, another antioxidant defense is to store and transport the metals in a form that cannot be used to produce free radicals. The mitochondria also produce enzymes that can repair the damage caused by free radicals.

Brain's susceptibility to oxidative stress

The brain is highly vulnerable to oxidative stress because it has a high energy demand, consumes a lot of oxygen, and is abundant in easily oxidized molecules and iron. Excessive free radicals trigger the detrimental chain reactions that damage the fats in the membranes of neurons, proteins that form the structure of brain cells and serve as enzymes, polysaccharides (sugar molecules bonded together that are the source of glucose), and DNA. Oxidative stress further leads to apoptosis, a process of controlled cell death that the body uses to eliminate damaged cells.

The brain also has very limited antioxidant defense systems. The CSF does not bind the metals to reduce their availability to oxidative actions. The brain's antioxidant system was found to decrease several-fold in people with mild cognitive impairment or Alzheimer's dementia than in adults with intact cognition.

Oxidative stress was shown to enhance BACE-1 and presinilin-1 activities, which lead to increased production of amyloid and tau hyperphosphorylation. Conversely, increased amyloid accumulation and tau hyperphosphorylation increase the production of free radicals and impair the antioxidant system.

Insulin Resistance and Glucose Hypometabolism

Glucose is, in fact, the sole fuel for the human brain, except during prolonged starvation, when the liver generates ketone bodies to partly replace glucose as fuel for the brain. The brain cannot use fatty acids as fuel because they are bound to albumin, a protein in the plasma and cannot cross the blood-brain barrier.

Brain's dependence on glucose

The brain cannot store fuel, so it needs a continuous supply of glucose. During rest, the brain consumes about 20% of the body's glucose. The brain uses 60% to 70% of the glucose to transmit nerve impulses and the rest for other essential brain activities such as synthesizing the neurotransmitters and their receptors to broadcast nerve impulses.

Brain cells receive glucose through glucose transporter protein with the help of insulin. Under normal conditions, Glucose transporter protein is saturated with glucose, so it gives a constant supply of glucose to the brain cells. Insulin is produced in the pancreas and transported by blood to the brain. Insulin can cross the blood-brain barrier to allow the brain cells use glucose as energy and modulate the survival of nerve cells, neurotransmission, and amyloid trafficking.

Impaired insulin signalling

Fluorodeoxyglucose PET studies show that the brain begins to use less glucose even before cognitive impairment appears. Decreased glucose use correlates with both the severity of cognitive impairment and AD hallmark brain changes. Insulin resistance and impaired insulin signaling have been identified as the main reasons why the brain uses less glucose.

Insulin resistance inhibits a brain cell's ability to use insulin effectively and can result from decreased insulin receptors. Impaired insulin signaling causes the excessive activation of glycogen synthase kinase-3β, an enzyme that reduces the availability of glucose to brain cells and the expression of glucose transporter proteins. Both excessive activation of glycogen synthase kinase-3β and decreased activity of glucose transporter proteins have been shown to increase amyloid deposition and tau hyperphosphorylation and vice versa.

Neuroinflammation

Neuroinflammation, a vital part of the brain's self-defense system, activates the brain's immune cells (microglia and astrocytes) to eliminate pathogens (such as bacteria and viruses) and cellular debris. Once they are eliminated, the inflammatory responses subside and eventually stop. However, if the inflammatory responses persist without resolution, such as in AD, they become problematic and can change, damage, or destroy neurons.

It remains unclear how neuroinflammation goes uncurbed in AD. Previously, neuroinflammation was thought to be caused by amyloid deposition. Recent evidence, however, suggests that neuroinflammation might occur independently of amyloid deposition. Mutations in genes that encode the production of cytokines, the inflammation biomarkers, have been found to increase the risk of AD and upregulate β-site APP cleaving enzyme 1 to increase amyloid production. Changes in microglia and astrocytes have also been found to affect synaptic formation and function.

Inflamm-aging

Neuroinflammation might result from inflamm-aging, a chronic, low-grade systemic inflammation linked with normal aging. Inflamm-aging is shown by high levels of cytokines such as interleukin-6, C-reactive protein, and tumor necrosis factor-α in the bloodstream. Blood cytokines "communicate" with the brain, as shown by the variation in brain structures in people with different levels of cytokines in the blood. Blood cytokine levels also reflect brain cytokine levels. Increased serum levels of interleukin-6 and C-reactive protein and decreased levels of interleukin-2 have been linked to poor cognitive performance.

Leaky gut

Leaky guts may be another cause of neuroinflammation and increased risk of AD. Leaky guts are increased permeability and/or decreased barrier function of the intestines. Leaky guts allow the foreign substances and pathogens that are normally blocked by the intestines to enter the bloodstream and cause systemic inflammation. Some of these foreign substances and pathogens may cross the blood-brain barrier to directly cause neuroinflammation in the brain.

Gut microbiome imbalance

Microbiome refers to the trillions of microorganisms such as bacteria, fungi, and other microbes that exist inside the intestines and on the skin. The gut microbiome begins to grow at birth when infants are exposed to the complex microorganisms in the vagina and continues to grow and diversify throughout life. It was estimated that there are 10 times more gut microorganisms than human cells. Most of the gut microbiome lives in a segment of the large intestine known as the caecum. There are more than 1,000 different species of gut microorganisms, which normally exist in balance. Gut bacteria have been studied more than other microorganisms. Some bacteria are known to cause diseases, while others have been found to be extremely important to the immune function, digestion, weight control, and overall health. As a result, the gut microbiome is often regarded as the "forgotten organ."

Recent large-scale studies such as the Human Microbiome Project have indicated that the gut microbiome might play a central role in gut-brain communication and brain function. The gut bacteria affect many functions of the body, producing substances such as tryptophan and short-chain fatty acids that can affect the brain. The gut bacteria can also generate neurotransmitters. Scientists are actively researching the role that microbiome plays in AD.

Vascular Dysfunction

The co-existence of vascular lesions and AD hallmark brain changes has long been seen in imaging studies. Vascular dysfunction is thought to contribute to AD in three ways: cerebral small vessel disease, shared cardiovascular conditions and risk factors, and shared abnormal changes of vascular dementia and AD.

Cerebral small vessel disease

Cerebral small vessel disease consists of many different conditions that affect the small arteries and microvessels (tiny blood vessels) of the brain and can be seen as white matter hyperintensity, cerebral microbleeds, or deep brain infarcts on brain imaging. Evidence supports the association between cerebral small vessel disease and AD hallmark brain changes, but the findings are mixed. The association also seems to be stronger in people with a certain genetic trait such as carriers of the apolipoprotein E gene allele 4.

Cerebral small vessel disease—and AD—are both common with advanced age. Hence, there is ongoing debate if cognitive impairment that increases with advanced age is the result of small vessel disease or AD separately or together.

Cardiovascular conditions and risk factors

Several cardiovascular conditions and risk factors for cerebrovascular disease and AD are shared, including high blood pressure, diabetes, high cholesterol, smoking, abnormal heart rhythm, and obesity. These risk factors have been linked to cognitive decline, onset of Alzheimer's dementia, and progression from mild cognitive impairment to Alzheimer's dementia. In particular, these risk factors in midlife, but not in late life, correlate with amyloid deposition. Treating cardiovascular risk factors have been shown to change the course of cognitive decline, and large-scale, international studies are underway.

High blood pressure. Chronic high blood pressure reduces cerebral blood flow to the gray matter and contributes to brain-blood barrier dysfunction, neuroinflammation, and amyloid deposition in AD-transgenic animal models. Greater amyloid load and shrinkage in the frontal cortex have been observed in people older than 70 years who had high blood pressure than those with normal blood pressure. Intensive control of high systolic blood pressure was recently found to reduce the risk of mild cognitive impairment by almost 20%.

Diabetes. Diabetes is a disease in which the body cannot make or respond to insulin adequately, so the body cannot use carbohydrates effectively. Diabetes is associated with reduced brain metabolism and hippocampal volume in older adults.

High cholesterol. High levels of cholesterol and homocysteine have been associated with AD brain changes in rodents. High cholesterol levels in the blood may also increase amyloid deposition and tau hyperphosphorylation; however, lipid-lowering drugs have not been found to produce cognitive benefits.

Abnormal heart rhythm. Atrial fibrillation, a type of abnormal heart rhythm, has been linked to AD. Abnormal heart rhythm is thought to affect blood supply to the brain, which contributes to cognitive decline.

Smoking. Smoking, particularly long-term smoking, induces oxidative stress in the brain. As previously mentioned, oxidative stress is an abnormal process that contributes to AD.

Obesity. Body mass index (BMI) is a measure of body fat and is calculated by dividing weight in kilograms by the square of height in meters. BMI is usually classified into four categories based on age and sex: normal, overweight, obese, or extremely obese. Generally speaking, BMI less than 18.5 is considered underweight, 18.5 to

24.9 normal, 25.0 to 29.9 overweight, and over 30 obese. Being overweight or obese in midlife has been linked with more severe neurofibrillary tangles and hippocampal shrinkage in old age.

Although different cardiovascular conditions and risk factors affect AD brain changes differently, they do share some common mechanisms of action. First, they decrease the structural elasticity and increase the stiffness of the arteries. The linkage between carotid arterial stiffness and amyloid deposition is strong in people with mild cognitive impairment and does not seem to differ by race or genotype. Arterial stiffness is thought to disrupt amyloid clearance from the brain and lead to amyloid deposition in blood vessel walls known as amyloid angiopathy. Amyloid angiopathy is consistently seen in 78% to 98% of the brains of people with Alzheimer's dementia on autopsy. Imaging studies have further shown that deterioration of the blood vessels precedes AD brain changes.

Second, cardiovascular conditions and risk factors reduce blood flow to the brain over time, resulting in chronic insufficient blood supply to the brain. Reduced cerebral blood flow occurs with aging but is substantially worse in people with Alzheimer's dementia in the frontal, temporal, and parietal lobes. Chronic insufficient blood supply to the brain is believed to speed up amyloid deposition and tau hyperphosphorylation and decrease glucose use in the brain.

Last, cardiovascular conditions and risk factors damage the blood-brain barrier based on imaging and postmortem studies. Because amyloid is cleared from the brain through the brain-blood barrier, a damage to the brain-blood barrier causes amyloid to build up in the brain.

Shared brain changes

The abnormal brain changes, such as neuroinflammation, mitochondrial dysfunction, and oxidative stress, are seen in both vascular dementia and AD. Vascular dementia and AD often co-exist, which gives rise to the term "mixed dementia." Untangling the relationship between these two types of dementia and the vascular contribution to AD are important areas of research.

Neurochemical Changes

AD hallmark and non-hallmark brain changes disturb the production and function of neurotransmitters in the brain. Neurotransmitters are the chemical messengers released to the synapses when nerve impulses arrive. Neurotransmitters then cross the synapses and are picked up by other neurons to advance the impulse.

AD changes a number of neurotransmitters that contribute to cognitive symptoms, including deficits in cholinergic neurotransmitters. Because reversing the cholinergic neurotransmitter deficits can be achieved by inhibiting the activities of the enzyme acetylcholinesterase, three of the five drugs that are approved by the FDA for AD treatment are acetylcholinesterase inhibitors: donepezil, rivastigmine tartrate, and galantamine hydrobromide.

Another biochemical change is excessive glutamate activity, which causes the over-stimulation of the N-methyl-D-aspartate receptors and damages neurons. The drug, memantine hydrochloride, protects the neurons by blocking the N-methyl-D-aspartate receptors from glutamate.

Other neurotransmitter deficits include deficiencies in GABAergic, noradrenergic, serotonergic, and perhaps dopaminergic neurotransmitters. While correcting the neurotransmitter deficits is an important area of AD research, drugs targeting neurotransmitter deficits do not alter AD hallmark brain changes. This is likely why these drugs have only limited, short-term effects on cognitive symptoms and cannot cure AD.

Infection

The quest for an infectious cause for AD traces back more than three decades. Several viruses and bacteria have been linked to AD, including *herpes simplex virus 1*, which causes oral herpes; *Chlamydophila pneumoniae*, which causes pneumonia and bronchitis; *spirochete*, which cause Lyme disease; *Treponema pallidum*, which causes syphilis; and *Porphyromonas gingivalis*, which triggers chronic gum disease. Some of these linkages are strong showing a fivefold increased prevalence of AD in people with Chlamydophila pneumoniae infection and a 10-fold increased prevalence in people with spirochetal infection.

Believers of the infectious origin of AD postulate that amyloid plaques and neurofibrillary tangles are the brain's attempts at isolating the infectious agent. When an infection occurs, it triggers neuroinflammation through a leaky blood-brain barrier in two ways. First, the viruses and bacteria get through to the brain more easily through the leaky blood-brain barrier to induce neuroinflammation. Second, the viruses and bacteria increase inflammation in the body by activating immune cells to produce inflammatory cytokines, and then the cytokines communicate with the brain or cross the blood-brain barrier to cause neuroinflammation. In contrast, doubters of the infectious origin of AD suggest that people affected AD simply were more likely to have these infections than those without AD and studies of the infectious origins of AD are methodologically flawed.

If an infection causes AD, then treating the infection could reduce the incidence of AD or alter its course. Research testing this hypothesis has produced mixed findings. For example, one study showed that AD occurred significantly less (up to 90%) in those who received herpes treatment than in those who did not. Another study reported that antibiotics such as doxycycline and rifampin reduced cognitive decline. However, other studies found no differences.

Apparently, more studies are needed to reveal the relationship between infection and AD.

In summary, AD brains show both the hallmark and non-hallmark changes which form a feedback loop to accelerate AD. It remains unknown what brain change(s) initiate AD. The clinical symptoms of AD may not appear until AD hallmark brain changes have reached a certain threshold that is yet unknown. The non-hallmark brain changes may lower this threshold, leading to earlier onset of cognitive decline. AD hallmark and non-hallmark brain changes interact in complex ways to affect different neural networks and contribute to varying symptom presentations and AD courses among individuals.

Key Messages

- AD imaging, CSF, and blood biomarkers have enabled the study of AD brain changes in living people and are classified using the AT(N) system.
- AD has two hallmark brain changes: amyloid plaques formed in the extracellular space and neurofibrillary tangles developed within the neurons.
- Amyloid-beta is produced from APP mainly by β- and γ-secretases in AD and its biomarkers include amyloid deposition on PET imaging and $A\beta_{42}$ and $A\beta_{42}/A\beta_{40}$ ratio in the CSF.
- In AD, tau becomes hyperphosphorylated, which disrupts the function of microtubules. Phosphorylated tau in the CSF and tau detected on tau PET are tau biomarkers.
- Neurodegeneration involves synaptic loss and neuronal injury and death. Its biomarkers include structural MRI changes and CSF total tau. Neurodegeneration is not a hallmark change of AD as it can be caused by other neurodegenerative conditions.

- Other AD non-hallmark brain changes include mitochondria dysfunction and oxidative stress, insulin resistance and glucose hypometabolism, neuroinflammation, vascular dysfunction, neurochemical changes, and infection.
- The brain is particularly vulnerable to oxidative stress due to its high use of energy and limited antioxidant defense system.
- Impaired insulin signaling causes the excessive activation of glycogen synthase kinase-3β and reduced expression of glucose transporter protein to reduce glucose use by the brain.
- Neuroinflammation seems to contribute to AD brain changes through inflamm-aging, leaky guts, and microbiome imbalance.
- Vascular dysfunction contributes to AD brain changes through cerebral small vessel diseases, cardiovascular conditions and risk factors, and vascular dementia.
- The ways that current AD drugs work is by correcting the neurotransmitter deficit or dysfunction.
- Infectious agents (e.g., *Herpes simplex virus 1, Chlamydophila pneumoniae, spirochete*, and *Porphyromonas gingivalis*) have been linked to AD.
- AD hallmark brain changes contribute to its non-hallmark brain changes and vice versa.

The Beginning Scenarios

Now that you have learned a great deal about AD disease processes, what are your thoughts on the discussions happened at the 2019 conference mentioned at the beginning of this chapter? What would you have said if you had been there? How would you explain AD brain changes if your family and friends asked you about them? What abnormal processes would you recommend the scientists to study in order to discover effective drug and non-drug treatments? It is no doubt that the brain changes in AD are complex.

The temporal relationship between AD hallmarks and non-hallmark changes remain unclear. All these brain changes interact in complex ways that are yet unknown and affect different people differently.

Chapter **3**

Who Is at Risk for Alzheimer's Disease?

*I*n August 2005, I completed the first year of my postdoctoral training at the Pennsylvania State University College of Nursing. That year was pivotal in helping me focus my career on the prevention and treatment of Alzheimer's disease (AD) using non-drug interventions to maximize functional independence and quality of life. I obtained some initial research funding to design and test an aerobic exercise program for older adults with Alzheimer's dementia. In the fall, I began to apply for an assistant professor position in research-intensive universities. As part of the job interview at a university, I taught a class to undergraduate nursing students about AD. When I asked who knew *someone with Alzheimer's dementia, only a few hands went up. Fast forward to fall 2014, when I gave a similar lecture at the University of Minnesota, most students raised their hands to this question. What do you think accounts for these different responses?*

In November 2016, I was invited to talk about my exercise research in AD at the University of Minnesota Center for Magnetic Resonance Research. After my presentation, a woman came up to thank me for doing this important work and shared her story. She grew up on a farm with five brothers and three sisters in Minnesota. Her father was diagnosed with Alzheimer's dementia at age 74 and passed away five years later. Her mother was diagnosed with Alzheimer's dementia at age 76 and had been living in a memory care unit since then. Her aunt on her father's side also had Alzheimer's dementia and died a couple of years ago in her 70s. "So, my siblings and I are all worried about our genetic risk for Alzheimer's," she said. "Now, thinking back, we believe that Mom and Dad started to have memory problems in their 60s. Because of my mom and aunt, my sisters and I are particularly concerned. Are women at a higher risk for Alzheimer's? Is there anything that we can do to better our odds?"

In December 2016, I traveled to Nanning, the capital of Guangxi Province in China, to meet with colleagues at the Guangxi Center for Disease Control and Prevention. The purpose of the trip was to plan the launch of a centenarian study funded by the University of Minnesota Academic Health Center Global Health Seed Grant. Of the 76 towns in China linked to longevity, 25 are in Guangxi. The number of centenarians living there had increased substantially, from 412 in 1982 to 2,977 in 2010. As part of the study planning, we visited three towns to meet some centenarians. They all appeared cognitively normal but had some mobility issues. Local health workers attributed it to diet (e.g., lack of meat, many grains and vegetables, 80% full stomach [due to limited food supplies]), lifelong farming practices, walking everywhere, and a natural environment.

As illustrated by the first scenario, AD has become a household word due to its prevalence and impact on people with Alzheimer's dementia, their families, and society at large. I am often approached by people who are concerned about their risk for AD, like the woman described in the second scenario.

In this chapter, you will learn why AD is everyone's business and how risk factors are identified. Then, you will become familiar with the risk and protective factors for AD that you can do something about, as well as those that you cannot change. As described in Chapter 1, AD is used to refer to the biologically abnormal brain process, while Alzheimer's dementia is the end phase of AD clinical manifestation after the preclinical AD and mild cognitive impairment due to AD phases.

Why Worry About Alzheimer's Dementia?

In Chapter 1, you learned that dementia is an umbrella term with many different causes and that AD is the most common cause. Dementia is the seventh leading cause of death globally. It is becoming less common in Europe and North America, but increasing in Asia. The number of people living with dementia will continue to rise because the older adult populations are growing. In 2018, the World Health Organization estimated that about 50 million people worldwide have dementia, 75 million people will have it by 2030, and 152 million will have it by 2050. Of the nearly 10 million people who develop dementia each year, 60% live in low- and middle-income countries.

Dementia is a major cause of loss of independence and disability and has significant physical, psychological, and economic impacts on people with dementia, their families, and society at large. The cost of medical, social, and informal caregiving for dementia exceeded $1 trillion in 2018 and will reach $2 trillion by 2030. In its *Global Action Plan on the Public Health Response to Dementia 2017–2025,* the World Health Organization recommends that countries conduct a dementia awareness or risk reduction campaign, develop a plan for caring for people with dementia, provide support and training to family and informal caregivers, and begin a dementia-friendly initiative.

Cost of Alzheimer's Dementia

In the United States, Alzheimer's dementia affected 5.7 million Americans in 2018, which is projected to reach 14 million in 2050. The number of new cases of Alzheimer's dementia will amount to 615,000 in 2030 and 959,000 in 2050. Someone develops Alzheimer's dementia every 65 seconds.

Alzheimer's dementia is the sixth leading cause of death for all ages and the fifth leading cause of death in older adults. One in three older adults dies from Alzheimer's dementia. People with Alzheimer's dementia are 61% more likely to die before age 80 than their peers who have intact cognition. In 2019, AD and related dementias cost the U.S. $290 billion and will cost about $1.1 trillion by 2050. An early, accurate diagnosis could save as much as $7.9 trillion in medical and caregiving expenses.

Impact on Family Caregivers

A family caregiver or a care partner is a family member, friend, or helper who takes care of another person. Caregiving may involve helping with activities of daily living such as paying bills, cooking, shopping, dressing, or toileting; providing emotional support; and meeting the health care needs such as preparing pills and driving to doctor's appointments.

In its *2019 Alzheimer's Facts and Figures,* the Alzheimer's Association estimated that 86% of the informal caregivers provided care for at least the past year; 57% have done so for four or more years, and more than 63% will continue to do so in the next five years. In 2019, each of 16 million informal caregivers provided about 22 hours of care per week, for 18.5 billion hours of unpaid care which was valued at more than $234 billion.

While caregiving is rewarding and induces positive feelings, it exerts heavy tolls on caregiver's well-being and health. Stress, depression, anxiety, and other mental health problems are more common in dementia caregivers than those who care for people with other conditions and non-caregivers. Informal caregiving is also linked to health decline, new symptoms and diseases, and worsening of existing conditions.

Outlook for a Cure for AD

Currently, no drug can prevent, slow, or cure AD. The U.S. Food and Drug Administration has approved five drugs to treat AD symptoms. Three drugs are cholinesterase inhibitors: Donepezil (approved in 1996 for all stages of Alzheimer's dementia), rivastigmine tartrate (approved in 1998 for mild to moderate Alzheimer's dementia), and galantamine hydrobromide (approved in 2001 for mild and moderate Alzheimer's dementia). The fourth drug, memantine hydrochloride (approved in 2003 for treating moderate and severe Alzheimer's dementia), is an N-methyl-D-aspartate receptor antagonist. The fifth drug is a combination of memantine and donepezil (approved in 2014 for moderate and severe Alzheimer's dementia).

From 2002 to 2012, more than 240 drugs were tested in at least 413 clinical trials. Unfortunately, 99.6% of them failed. The only drug that was successful was memantine. Some recent, very promising trials of humanized monoclonal amyloid antibodies also had disappointing results. Other promising drugs are currently in clinical trials.

AD Prevention as a Priority

It is no doubt that preventing AD is a public health priority. A 12-month delay in the onset of Alzheimer's dementia could reduce the number of people with it by 9.2 million, while a five-year delay could prevent 57% of AD cases. This means that the 10.5% lifetime risk for Alzheimer's dementia in 65 years old would be reduced to 5.7%. Hence, extensive efforts have been devoted to developing and testing both drug and non-drug treatments to prevent AD, including our work in aerobic exercise and cognitive training. Moreover, the brain is plastic and can compensate for the damage caused by AD, especially during preclinical AD and mild cognitive impairment phases. The level of plasticity extenuates as AD progresses from mild to severe stages of Alzheimer's dementia.

What Are the Risk Factors for AD?

Risk factors predict the onset and progression of a disease and provide the targets for developing treatments. One way to think about risk factors is to classify them as modifiable and non-modifiable. Modifiable risk factors are changeable, so you can take actions to reduce your risk. Modifiable risk factors for AD include cardiovascular conditions and risk factors (e.g., diabetes, high blood pressure, high cholesterol, obesity, and smoking), traumatic brain injury, low educational level, and behavioral and psychological symptoms (e.g., parkinsonism, apathy, anxiety, depression, and sleep disturbances). It is estimated that as many as a third of all AD cases might be caused by these modifiable risk factors.

Another common phrase you may have heard of is protective factors that protect against the development of a disease and/or can slow down the progression of a disease. Risk factors and protective factors are, in a sense, two sides of the same coin, if they, in essence, are referring to the same thing. For example, physical inactivity is a risk factor for AD, so its flip side, physical activity, is a protective factor. To avoid listing both sides of the same coin in this chapter, only one side is listed based on the research tradition. Protective factors for AD include physical activity, brain or cognitive reserve, cognitive and social activities, and a heart-healthy diet (Figure 3.1).

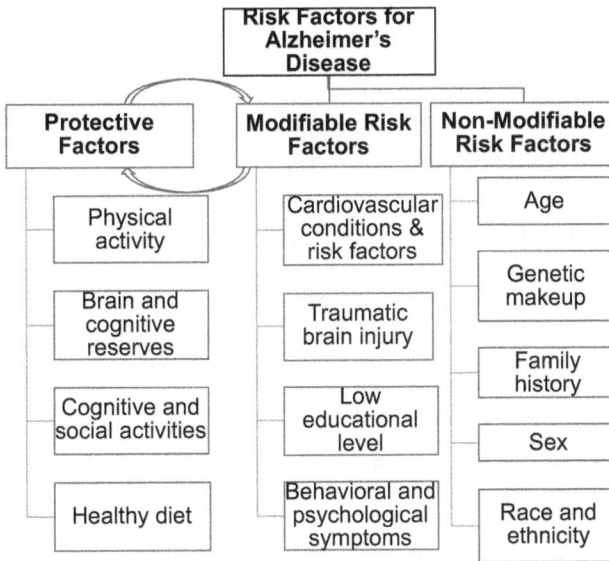

Figure 3.1. Risk and Protective Factors for Alzheimer's Disease

Non-modifiable risk factors, in contrast, are what you were born with (e.g., age, genetic makeup, family history, sex, and race and ethnicity), so you may not be able to do anything about them. Although gender transformation is doable, there are insufficient data to know if such a transformation alters AD risk. One day, genetic editing may become a standard treatment for AD, so genetic risk may also become modifiable, but it is not yet an option. Given these, gender and genetics are described as non-modifiable risk factors in this chapter.

Figure 3.1 depicts the well-established risk factors for AD at a glance. Recent evidence suggests that hearing loss is a risk factor for AD as well.

Having one or more risk factors does not guarantee that you will develop Alzheimer's dementia in your lifetime. The onset and symptoms of AD are highly variable among people. As you have read in Chapter 2, multiple abnormal changes occur in AD and interact in complex ways that are not yet understood. A single or even multiple risk factors, modifiable or not, may not be enough to cause AD. An exception is when you have the genes for early-onset or familial AD described later in this chapter.

What Are the Modifiable Risk Factors for AD?

The evidence on modifiable risk factors for AD is still evolving. Some factors have been well-studied, while others have not. Please be reminded that some risk factors are not discussed here because their flip sides have traditionally been studied in research and are covered under protective factors. Now, let us first review what is known about each risk factor.

Cardiovascular Conditions and Risk Factors

The word "cardiovascular" means heart- and blood vessel-related. Factors that negatively affect the health of heart and blood vessels strongly influence brain health. The human brain makes up about 2% of the bodyweight but uses 20% of the oxygen and energy supplies. Thus, healthy heart and blood vessels are important to ensure that oxygen and energy reach the brain. From this perspective, it should not be surprising that cardiovascular conditions and risk factors such as diabetes, high blood pressure, high cholesterol, obesity, smoking, and a poor diet increase the risk for AD.

An interesting finding is that the timing of cardiovascular risk factors seems to count. Cardiovascular conditions and risk factors in midlife have been associated with an increased risk for AD. Type 2 diabetes in midlife has been linked to a 50% to 58% higher risk for mild cognitive impairment. Midlife pre-high blood pressure (systolic blood pressure 120 to 139 mm Hg or diastolic pressure 80 to 89 mm Hg) and high blood pressure (systolic blood pressure above 139 mm Hg or diastolic pressure above 89 mm Hg) have been linked to a 40% to 140% increased risk for AD. Midlife high cholesterol has been linked to about a 45% higher risk for mild cognitive impairment. Being overweight in midlife has been associated with one or twofold increased risk for dementia, while obesity increases the risk by five to sevenfold. Compared with nonsmokers, smokers have a 1.45- to twofold higher rate for AD. A long smoking history doubles the risk for mild cognitive impairment.

In contrast, obesity and high blood pressure after age 80 have been linked to a decreased risk for AD. It is unclear why, but these conditions in late life probably compensate for the loss of brain blood supply or defend against other diseases to meet the oxygen and energy demands of the brain.

Traumatic Brain Injury

Traumatic brain injury has gained substantial attention in its linkage to AD with some studies reporting it as the strongest risk factor for AD. Traumatic brain injury refers to a sudden trauma to the brain through an abrupt and forceful collision with an object, a whiplash-like incident, or an object that pierces the skull and damages the brain tissue. Traumatic brain injury is staged as mild, moderate, or severe based on either the duration of symptoms (loss of consciousness and posttraumatic memory loss) or scores on the 15-point Glasgow Coma Scale.

- Mild: Loss of consciousness or posttraumatic memory loss of fewer than 30 minutes or an initial score of 13 to 15 on the Glasgow Coma Scale. Mild traumatic brain injury is the most common type and makes up about 75% of all traumatic brain injuries. It is also known as a concussion.
- Moderate: Loss of consciousness or posttraumatic memory loss of 30 minutes to 24 hours or an initial score of nine to 12 on the Glasgow Coma Scale.
- Severe Loss of consciousness or posttraumatic memory loss of at least 24 hours or an initial score of eight or less on the Glasgow Coma Scale.

According to the U.S. Centers for Disease Control and Prevention, about 1.7 million Americans suffer from traumatic brain injury in any given year. Traumatic brain injury is estimated to affect 17% to 22% of military personnel, with blast injury the most common cause. In civilians, the leading causes of traumatic brain injury are falls, object strikes, and motor vehicle accidents. Falls contribute to more than two-thirds of traumatic brain injuries in older adults living at home.

About 56% of people with traumatic brain injury show cognitive impairment that meets the criteria for Alzheimer's dementia. The more severe the traumatic brain injury, the higher the risk for dementia, especially in people with the apolipoprotein (*APOE*) gene allele 4 (ε4) variant. Mild traumatic brain injury is often unrecognized but can increase the risk for AD twofold. traumatic brain injury has also been linked to increased amyloid precursor protein and diffuse amyloid plaques in some cases. Some studies have reported that traumatic brain injury is associated with a 60% increased risk for dementia over nine years in veterans, with the risk increasing two to fourfold decades after traumatic brain injury. However, other studies have found neither increased risk nor increased AD biomarkers in veterans with traumatic brain injury, which might be attributable to small sample sizes.

Low Educational Level

Low educational level has been associated with an increased risk for AD and fast AD progression. However, isolating the relationship between education and AD is difficult, because other factors might explain their association. For example, people with low educational level might work in jobs that are less cognitively challenging, have more cardiovascular diseases and risk factors, and have a lower socioeconomic status that limits access to nutritious foods and adequate medical care than people with high educational level.

Behavioral and Psychological Symptoms

Apathy, anxiety, depression, sleep disturbances, and Parkinsonism have been linked to an increased risk for mild cognitive impairment and Alzheimer's dementia. These symptoms also seem to predict the progression from mild cognitive impairment to Alzheimer's dementia.

Apathy

Apathy refers to a reduction in voluntary, goal-directed cognition, action, and emotion. It has been strongly linked to progression from mild cognitive impairment to Alzheimer's dementia. Among people with amnestic mild cognitive impairment as the presenting symptom, apathy increases the risk of progression to Alzheimer's dementia seven times.

Anxiety

Anxiety refers to excessive fear or worries and other symptoms (restlessness, fatigue, difficulty concentrating, irritability, muscle tension, and sleep disturbances). In older adults who had normal cognition, anxiety is associated with reduced episodic memory and executive function as well as an increased risk for mild cognitive impairment and progression to Alzheimer's dementia. Anxiety is also related to high levels of amyloid deposition and temporal lobe shrinkage.

Depression

Depression is marked by sadness and loss of interest in usual activities. Older adults with depression perform worse on tests of episodic memory, executive function, and language. Depression has been linked to about twofold increased risk for mild cognitive impairment and accelerated cognitive decline. People with depression have more than 50% higher risk for Alzheimer's dementia and a faster cognitive decline than those without depression.

Depression was reported to cause about 10% of Alzheimer's dementia cases worldwide. Depression may act either as a state preceding cognitive decline or an early sign of Alzheimer's dementia. Depression in midlife and late life has been linked to an increased amyloid burden and a small hippocampus. Some studies suggest that severe depressive symptoms predict and double the risk of progression from mild cognitive impairment to Alzheimer's dementia, but other studies have not found such a relationship.

Sleep disturbances

Individuals with sleep disturbances have a 1.68 times higher risk for cognitive impairment or Alzheimer's dementia. Short (less than seven hours) and long (more than eight hours) duration of sleep per night, poor sleep efficiency, and circadian rhythm abnormalities have been linked to an increased risk for Alzheimer's dementia. Melatonin levels decrease in the cerebrospinal fluid in people with preclinical AD, suggesting that the reduction may be either an early marker or cause of Alzheimer's dementia. Sleep disorders such as excessive daytime sleepiness and obstructive sleep apnea have also been linked to amyloid accumulation in the brain.

Parkinsonism

Parkinsonism symptoms include rigidity, shuffling gait, slow movements, and tremors. The incidence of Alzheimer's dementia seems higher in people with these symptoms. Parkinsonism also accelerates the progression of AD to disability and death.

Dispelling Myths

Environmental toxins and metal accumulations have attracted a lot of attention as the risk factors for AD, including aluminum or mercury poisoning. Currently, the evidence does not support the link between aluminum or mercury poisoning and AD. Geography has also been examined because a high number of cases of Alzheimer's dementia has been reported in rural areas. However, geographic differences may be explained by the low educational level or socioeconomic status and difference in AD diagnosis and identification methods.

What Are the Protective Factors for AD?

The protective factors for AD include physical activity, brain and cognitive reserves, cognitive and social activities, and a heart-healthy diet. While the strengths of evidence vary depending on the factor, authoritative agencies such as the National Academy of Medicine consider the overall evidence strong enough to make a recommendation.

Physical Activity

The linkage between physical activity and AD risk has been evaluated by at least 17 prospective longitudinal studies with more than 21 cohorts of 357 to 4,406 participants. These studies commonly compared vigorous or moderate physical activity with low or no physical activity. Because of the sheer number of studies and cohorts, the findings are inconsistent, showing no to large risk reduction for AD from physical activity. Similar findings are also found between physical activity and dementia of any type (more than 25 studies with more than 30 cohorts of 147 to 4,761 participants). Taken together, the overall results indicate that moderate to vigorous physical activity is linked to a reduced risk for Alzheimer's dementia and dementia of any type.

Another way to make sense of a large body of individual studies is through systematic reviews and meta-analyses. Systematic reviews are a type of literature review that uses a systematic method to identify individual studies on a topic of interest, critically assesses each study for quality and risk of bias, and synthesizes their study findings to draw conclusions. If a systematic review further employs a statistical method to pool together data from the individual studies to re-analyze them, then it becomes a meta-analysis.

The number of systematic reviews and meta-analyses on physical activity and Alzheimer's dementia has also grown substantially. Now, you might sigh and ask if this means that the findings are again inconsistent. Unfortunately, yes. Recent meta-analyses that have used better methods and had low publication bias report that high physical activity is linked to an average 38% risk reduction for Alzheimer's dementia (range from 25% to 51%). Moderate physical activity is linked to an average 29% risk reduction for Alzheimer's dementia (range from 11% to 44%). A sex difference has also been reported. Men seem to experience more risk reduction from physical activity (39%) than women (36%).

Similar findings were found between physical activity and dementia of any type. When compared with no or low physical activity, high physical activity was associated with a risk reduction of, on average, 21% for dementia of any type (ranging from 6% to 39%) and a 33% risk reduction for cognitive decline (ranging from

22% to 45%). The risk reduction for moderate physical activity was, on average, 24% for dementia of any type (ranging from 12% to 31% and 26% for cognitive decline (ranging from 10% to 40%). Unlike Alzheimer's dementia, the risk reduction for dementia of any type only slightly favors men (23%) over women (22%). In contrast, women seem to have more risk reduction for cognitive decline (35%) than men (29%).

People with Alzheimer's or other dementias appear to be less physically active than peers without dementia. Because AD can last for years or decades before any noticeable symptoms, AD brain changes can make people less motivated or interested in physical activity. As the brain changes progress, people are less and less physically active and eventually stop or are unable to perform physical activity on their own. As a result, AD and reduced physical activity form a vicious, downward spiral in which increased AD brain changes lead to reduced physical activity. Reduced physical activity, in turn, contributes to more AD brain changes. Hence, increasing physical activity breaks this vicious cycle.

Brain and Cognitive Reserves

Chapters 1 and 2 mentioned two discrepancies in the pathogenic process of AD and the clinical diagnosis of Alzheimer's dementia. The first is the lack of symptoms in some people with extensive AD brain changes. The second occurs in some people who had relatively few AD brain changes but extensive AD symptoms.

One reason for these discrepancies is brain and cognitive reserves. Brain reserve refers to the brain's ability to tolerate injury with showing no or few symptoms of cognitive impairment. Cognitive reserve is the brain's ability to compensate for injury using alternative brain networks or cognitive strategies.

Brain reserve and cognitive reserve are often used interchangeably because their difference is not clear-cut. One way to distinguish them is that brain reserve speaks from a biological or structural perspective. A large brain reserve means a large number of healthy neurons and dense synapses. Cognitive reserve, on the other hand, is used more from a functional perspective and represents the brain's ability to mobilize alternative networks or strategies to cope with the damage. A large brain reserve likely supports a large cognitive reserve because they are influenced by similar factors.

A large brain or cognitive reserve has a protective effect on cognition and is linked to a reduced risk for AD. Although a large brain or cognitive reserve allows people to tolerate AD brain changes for a longer period of time, the protective effect of the brain or cognitive reserve on cognition is likely not linear. Once the reserve is "maxed out" or reaches a "tipping point," a rapid cognitive decline can occur afterward.

Cognitive and Social Activities

Cognitively challenging or stimulating activities, as well as social activities, have been linked to a reduced risk for AD. Examples of these activities include participating in cognitive training, learning new things, playing mental games, and increased job complexity, social engagement, and social interaction. These activities, along with education and socioeconomic status, are all believed to increase brain and cognitive reserves.

Computerized cognitive training has been found to produce large improvements in cognition which can last after the training period is over. Cognitive training increases the functional connectivity in critical brain networks as captured by imaging studies. It appears that 10–20 hours of cognitive training are sufficient to generate cognitive benefits in older adults with mild cognitive impairment. It remains unknown how many or how much social activities are needed to reduce AD risk.

Healthy Diet

A heart-healthy diet is important to cardiovascular health. A heart-healthy diet is composed of fruits, vegetables, fish, chicken, whole grains, nuts, legumes, and limited saturated fats, red meat, and sugar. Examples of heart-healthy diets are the Mediterranean or Dietary Approaches to Stop Hypertension (DASH) diet. Both diets have been linked to improved cognition and a 2% to 40% risk reduction for AD. A heart-healthy diet may protect against AD by promoting cardiovascular function and curbing oxidative stress and neuroinflammation, the non-hallmark AD brain changes as described in Chapter 2.

High levels of vitamin E in the blood are linked to a reduced risk for AD. However, clinical trials of vitamin E supplements have not succeeded, which may be attributable to the use of only one form of vitamin E, α-tocopherol, and the lack of measurement of participants' vitamin E level (low or normal) before the trials started. There are eight forms of vitamin E. Some studies show that high serum levels of γ-tocopherol and β-tocotrienol, total tocopherols, and total tocotrienols—not α-tocopherol—are linked to a reduced risk for AD.

Another dietary supplement under investigation is a bacteria "cocktail" to rebalance gut microbiome and fix leaky guts. Better guts can prevent foreign substances and materials from entering the bloodstream and causing inflammation, particularly neuroinflammation. Human studies of microbiome cocktails are underway to test their effects on AD prevention and treatment.

Other Modifiable Factors

Adequate management of cardiovascular conditions and risk factors, as well as behavioral and psychological symptoms, likely helps to promote brain health. Strategies to avoid traumatic brain injury are important for protecting against Alzheimer's dementia.

Studies of multipronged lifestyle changes to address multiple cardiovascular conditions and risk factors have had some exciting initial findings, and large trials are in progress.

Environmental changes to reduce falls and traumatic brain injury include a well-lit physical environment that is free of tripping hazards such as throw rugs. Always wear a seatbelt, and wear a helmet when riding a bicycle, snowmobile, or other vehicles that are open or do not have restraints.

While getting more education could protect against AD, there may be a ceiling to this benefit. Some findings suggest that the protective effect of education may begin to taper off after high school. Recently, hearing loss was linked to Alzheimer's dementia, but more research is needed to confirm if improving hearing is beneficial for reducing the risk for Alzheimer's dementia.

What Are the Non-Modifiable Risk Factors?

Age, genetic risk, and having a family history of AD are the non-modifiable risk factors for AD. None of these factors by itself is sufficient to cause AD except for certain genes, and just because you have these risk factors, you are not guaranteed to get AD.

Age

Age is the single most important risk factor for AD because the vast majority of Alzheimer's dementia cases occur in people 65 years old and older. The risk for Alzheimer's dementia differs among age groups—young-old (65 to 74 years), middle-old (75 to 84), and the oldest-old (85 and older). The prevalence of Alzheimer's dementia doubles for every five-year increase in age. AD affects about 1%–3% of the young-old group, 17% of the middle-old group, and 32% to 48% of the oldest-old group. The oldest-old group is the fastest-growing segment of the older adult population. In the United States, the oldest-old group comprised 14%

of the older adult population in 2012 and is projected to rise to 22% by 2050.

About 80% of dementia occurs in older adults 75 years old and older. The incidence of dementia continues to increase after age 90, but the rate of increase seems to slow or plateau afterward. The prevalence of dementia is 45% to 70% in centenarians. About 30% of centenarians do not have dementia, re-affirming that dementia is not a normal part of aging. People with Alzheimer's dementia at a younger age live longer than those whose dementia started at an older age.

Genetic Risk

A genetic risk refers to a certain gene or mutation in a gene that increases the risk of disease. A mutation is a change in the structure of a gene. Based on the genetic risk and age of onset, AD has traditionally been classified into two types: early-onset AD and late-onset AD. Early-onset AD is also called young-onset, autosomal dominant, or familial AD and mainly affects people younger than 65 years of age and even in their 20s and 30s. In contrast, Late-onset AD occurs in people 65 and older and is used to be called sporadic AD, but not much anymore. Other than indicating the different genetic risk and age of onset, the distinction between early-onset and late-onset AD is not very useful because AD brain changes are similar for both.

Genetic risk for Early-Onset AD

Some early-onset AD cases are caused by an inherited mutation in one of three genes, including the amyloid precursor protein (*APP*) gene located on chromosome 21, presenilin 1 (*PSEN-1*) gene on chromosome 14, presenilin 2 (*PSEN-2*) gene on chromosome 1. These genes are named after the proteins they encode. Some early-onset AD cases may be related to other genetic mutations such as three chromosomes 21 in Down syndrome, *PSD2*, *TCIRG1*, *RIN3,* and so on.

People with mutations in the *PSEN-1* and *APP* genes are destined to develop early-onset AD, while those with mutations in the *PSEN-2* gene have a 95% chance of developing early-onset AD. Mutations in these genes increase the amyloid production and accumulation in the brain. In individuals with mutations in these genes, the onset of mild cognitive impairment is most likely due to AD. However, if and when they will progress from mild cognitive impairment to Alzheimer's dementia is highly variable. Having a first-degree relative with Alzheimer's dementia, however, does not necessarily mean you have a mutation in these genes and will develop EOAD.

People with Down syndrome have an extra copy of chromosome 21, which contains the *APP* gene. The extra copy may cause an increased production of amyloid starting at birth, but the precise mechanism is unclear. People with Down syndrome get amyloid plaques as early as 12 years old. By age 40, most of them develop the classic amyloid plaques and neurofibrillary tangles in their brains and about 30% have early-onset AD in their 50s.

Genetic risk for Late-Onset AD

The causes of late-onset AD are not completely understood but likely include a combination of genetic, environmental, and lifestyle factors. The best-known genetic risk factor is the *APOE* gene which encodes apolipoprotein E on chromosome 19. The *APOE* gene is implicated in impaired amyloid metabolism, transport, and clearance. Every person has two alleles (meaning alternative forms and being noted with "ε") of the *APOE* gene by inheriting one from each parent. There are six different ε combinations as ε2/ε2, ε2/ε3, ε2/ε4, ε3/ε3, ε3/ε4, and ε4/ε4. More than half of the population have ε3/ε3 and about 14% have ε3/ε4 or ε4/ε4, but these estimates vary by studies, countries, and race/ethnicity.

Compared with the neutral ε3/ε3 combination, having the ε2/ε2 is associated with a decreased risk for late-onset AD. Having one ε4 increases the risk for late-onset AD three to fourfold and having two ε4 increases the risk five to 18-fold. Among people with late-onset AD, about 56% to 65% have at least one ε4 and roughly 11% have two ε4. Having the ε4 copy may lower the age of AD onset by six to seven years. The Genome-Wide Association Study has linked many other genes to late-onset AD such as TREM2, PICALM, and BIN1. Some of these genes such as TREM2 are predominantly expressed in microglia, the supporting cells of the brain, which suggests that microglia may play an important role in AD brain changes.

Family History

Having a first-degree relative such as a parent with Alzheimer's dementia increases a person's lifetime risk for Alzheimer's dementia to about 37%, compared with a 10% to 20% risk in the general population. Having two parents with Alzheimer's dementia increases the risk to 31% to 54%.

There is certainly a potential genetic component at play because first-degree relatives share similar genetic makeup; however, it does not necessarily mean that they have mutations in the *APP*, *PSEN-1*, or *PSEN-2* genes. The increased risk cannot be entirely explained by having the same *APOE* forms either.

A recent study suggested that having an extended family member with Alzheimer's dementia increases a person's risk, even when the first-degree relatives did not have it. People with three or four relatives with Alzheimer's dementia were more than twice likely to develop AD.

Sex

In the United States, about two-thirds of people with Alzheimer's dementia are women; however, sex differences in Alzheimer's dementia have not been consistently reported. Some studies show a higher prevalence of Alzheimer's dementia in women than men, while others suggest no differences. One estimate suggests 20% and 10% lifetime risk for Alzheimer's dementia in American women and men who are 45 years old, respectively.

The sex difference in Alzheimer's dementia was initially thought to be artificial because women, on average, live longer than men, and age is the single greatest risk factor for Alzheimer's dementia. In addition, middle-aged men have more cardiovascular conditions and risk factors and higher rates of death from cardiovascular diseases than women; hence, men who survive into old age may have few cardiovascular conditions and risk factors. In contrast, women start to lose the protective cardiovascular benefits from hormones as they enter menopause and become susceptible to cardiovascular conditions in old age. Vascular dysfunction is a non-hallmark AD brain changes as described in Chapter 2. In recent years, possible sex-specific biological mechanisms have drawn considerable attention and seem to indicate that there is indeed a differential risk for AD by sex. Male and female brains are built a bit differently. Female brains seem to contain high levels of certain proteins that predispose them to AD than male brains.

Race and Ethnicity

Alzheimer's dementia has been found to be more prevalent in African and Hispanic Americans than white Americans, but it is unknown if there are true race and ethnicity differences. Socioeconomic factors, education, and other risk factors may be the reasons.

In summary, this chapter covers the most common risk factors for AD but is not intended to be all-inclusive because risk identification is an evolving field of research with new emerging evidence. Quantifying the risk for AD can be difficult because research findings vary depending on the study location, population, and methods. Studies are underway to examine the mechanism of action of a factor, modification of multiple risk factors, and innovative method such as machine learning on AD risk prediction and reduction. The unique combination of risk factors in each person at least partially explains why the onset and progression of AD vary so much among people.

Key Messages

- Dementia is a global crisis and a major cause of disability and death with tremendous social and financial impacts.
- The lifetime risk for Alzheimer's dementia at age 45 is about 20% in American women and about 10% in American men.
- Risk factors are classified as modifiable if they can be changed through lifestyle modification and treatment and non-modifiable if they cannot. Protective factors are, in a way, the flip side of modifiable risk factors.
- Modifiable risk factors for Alzheimer's dementia include cardiovascular conditions and risk factors, traumatic brain injury, low educational level, and behavioral and psychological symptoms.
- Protective factors against Alzheimer's dementia include physical activity, brain and cognitive reserves, cognitive activities, social activities, and a heart-healthy diet.
- Non-modifiable risk factors for Alzheimer's dementia include age, genetic mutation, family history of Alzheimer's dementia, sex, race, and ethnicity.
- Having one or more risk factors for AD does not mean that an individual will develop Alzheimer's dementia in his or her lifetime. Multiple risk factors likely act together in complex ways to affect AD onset and progression.

The Beginning Scenarios

Now, you have learned about the impact of Alzheimer's dementia and its risk factors. Let us go back to the scenarios introduced at the beginning of this chapter. How do you explain the different responses students gave to the same question about if they knew someone with Alzheimer's dementia? The essence of this story is that Alzheimer's dementia has become a household phrase due to public health efforts to address this epidemic. Even if you do not know anyone with Alzheimer's dementia, chances are that you know someone who knows a person with Alzheimer's dementia.

How would you answer the questions posed by the woman who attended my presentation at the University of Minnesota Center for Magnetic Resonance Research? Two of her first-degree relatives (both parents) have Alzheimer's dementia, so she has a family history of it. The risk for Alzheimer's dementia for her and her siblings is much higher than that for someone with no or only one first-degree relative with dementia. She may or may not have *APOE* ε4 though. I discussed with her a number of things that she and her siblings can do to better their odds, such as working with their health care providers on regular assessments of cognition, control of any existing medical conditions, participation in physical activity (particularly aerobic exercise), cognitive training, social engagement, heart-healthy diet, weight management, stress reduction, and better sleep.

How have the risk and protective factors for Alzheimer's dementia been at play in the centenarians in Guangxi Province, China? Do you feel puzzled because they are free of Alzheimer's dementia despite lacking education and having advanced age? Or did you breathe a sigh of relief because you are assured that having a few risk factors is really not the end of the world? The moral of the story is that you may never develop Alzheimer's dementia, even if the odds are against you.

Chapter 4

What Is Exercise?

One day my neighbor said, "Fang, you are amazing!" "Why? What did I do?" I asked. "You were stretching your leg above your head on the tree." "Oh, that was not me. It was my mom." My neighbor was dumbfounded, and we both laughed. My mom was in her late 60s then and a strong believer in exercising her way to health and longevity. Her daily exercise routine includes at least an hour of walking around the neighborhood and another hour of stretching poses such as propping her leg up on the tree trunk in our backyard.

I became close with a colleague when we began to work together on Alzheimer's research. Through the processes of writing papers and grant proposals, we found that we really liked each other as *professional career women. At her suggestion, we signed up for an employee fitness program at the University of Minnesota as something to do together outside of work. The fitness program involves an hour of muscle-building exercise using an exercise ball. It was perfect because a few months ago, my primary care provider had recommended it. Since then, I have been doing this type of exercise about twice a week.*

One day, I was invited to talk about my research on aerobic exercise in older adults with Alzheimer's dementia at the Walker Art Center in Minneapolis, MN, where I met another speaker. This speaker operates a tai chi studio in St Paul. She discussed the rationale behind tai chi and guided us in practicing some basic movements.

Given that I am from China, it is very natural for my colleagues to consult with me on their trips to China. On their return, they often marvel at the activities, such as square dances, in parks and city centers. Square dancing with different levels of physical exertion and choreographic complexity has become a national sensation, particularly in women. In fact, there are local and national square dance competitions. Some women have danced to prominence in the international media. Every time I visit China, I square dance after dinner whenever possible.

One day, I was chatting with a woman who served on a community committee with me in Saint Paul. She retired several years ago. When I asked her how she spends her days in retirement, she said that she attends different group fitness classes at the University of Minnesota Recreation and Wellness Center. The classes include Zumba, yoga, high-intensity interval training, and cycling, just to name a few. Most of her classmates are college students. She laughed when she noted that the classes seemed easy for them and that she was the only one huffing and puffing. "How do you feel then?" I asked. "It has been fun," she said. "I am highly motivated to perform."

Can you tell personal stories about your own experience with exercise? I bet you can and that your stories are probably more interesting than mine. The purpose of my stories is to give you a peek into the variety of exercises available to you. Each scenario above presents a different type of exercise. If you cannot name the types of exercise, do not worry; you will be able to after you read this chapter.

In this chapter, you will discover the difference between physical activity and exercise and the different types of exercises and their respective effects on physical fitness. Next, you will find out age-related changes in physical activity and fitness, as well as the risks and health benefits of exercise. Last, you will become familiar with the exercise recommendations for older adults.

How Do Physical Activity and Exercise Differ?

The terms "physical activity" and "exercise" are often used synonymously, but they are not the same. Physical activity is a broader term than exercise and includes both exercise and non-exercise physical activity. The American College of Sports Medicine defines physical activity as "the bodily movement that is produced by the contraction of skeletal muscles and that substantially increases energy expenditure." The World Health Organization has a similar definition for physical activity: "any bodily movement produced by skeletal muscles that require energy expenditure."

Exercise is a type of physical activity and refers to "the planned, structured, and repetitive bodily movement done to improve or maintain one or more components of physical fitness," according to the American College of Sports Medicine.

Non-exercise or leisure-time physical activity refers to activities embedded in your daily life. Examples include household work such as cooking, cleaning, dishwashing, and doing laundry; home repairs such as fixing a broken pipe, painting, and changing a lightbulb; yard work such as mowing a lawn, gathering leaves, and plowing snow; and recreational activities such as fishing and hunting.

What Are the Different Types of Exercise?

Although there are other ways to categorize exercise, it is usually classified into four types: aerobic, strength, balance, and flexibility. Each type improves or maintains some specific aspects of physical fitness.

Aerobic Exercise

Aerobic exercise involves continuous, rhythmic movements of body parts (e.g., legs, arms) that provide cardiorespiratory conditioning. The term "aerobic" means "with oxygen," indicating that the respiratory and cardiovascular systems control the amount of oxygen delivered to the muscles to help them burn fuel and move. Aerobic exercise is also known as cardiorespiratory or endurance exercise.

Aerobic exercise is often labeled based on its impact on the musculoskeletal system. High-impact aerobic exercise, which results in both feet coming off the ground at the same time, includes running, jumping rope, and step aerobics. Low-impact aerobic exercise, which is often performed on exercise equipment in fitness centers and rehabilitation settings, includes swimming, walking, elliptical training, total body recumbent stepping, cycling on a cycle ergometer, and rowing. Aerobic exercise mainly improves aerobic fitness and body composition but can improve all other aspects of physical fitness, particularly in people who are physically deconditioned and older adults.

Strength Exercise

Strength exercise causes the muscles to contract against external resistance to increase strength, muscle mass, and muscle endurance. Strength exercise is also called muscle building, weight lifting, and resistance exercise. External resistance can come from a variety of strength-building machines, low-cost alternatives such as free weights and rubber exercise tubing or bands, household items such as bricks or jugs of water, or simply one's own body weight. Resistance exercise is best known for its positive effects on bones, muscles, connective tissues, strength, insulin sensitivity, and body composition.

Balance Exercise

Balance exercise, or neuromuscular exercise, focuses on challenging balance and proprioception—awareness of one's position and movement. During the past few decades, there has been an increase in the popularity of non-Western styles of exercise that fall in this category, including qigong, yoga, and tai chi. These forms of exercise build on meditative movement and can be more enjoyable. The dynamic movements and isometric muscle contractions of these exercises have been shown to increase muscular strength and joint range of motion, particularly in novices, people who are deconditioned, and older adults.

Flexibility Exercise

Flexibility exercise, or stretching, extends a body part such as a limb. It is an important but often neglected part of an exercise program. Stretching is particularly important for maintaining postural stability, preventing and managing nonspecific low back pain, and slowing an age-related decline in joint range of motion and loss of skeletal muscle elasticity.

A variety of exercises are available for each type of exercise. Some examples are provided in Table 4.1.

Table 4.1. Examples of the Four Types of Exercises

Aerobic	Resistance	Balance	Flexibility
Walking	Free weights	Yoga	Stretching
Jogging	Weight machines	Tai Chi	Yoga
Swimming	Medicine balls	Stability	Tai Chi
Rowing	Resistance bands	exercises	Pilates
Biking	Some Tai Chi	One leg stands	
Rope skipping	Some yoga	Bosu ball	
Dancing	Pilates		
Water aerobics	Circuit training		

How Does Exercise Affect Physical Fitness?

Physical fitness is an umbrella term with five components: aerobic fitness, muscular fitness, body composition, balance, and flexibility. As mentioned previously, exercise is a form of physical activity designed to improve aspects of physical fitness.

Aerobic Fitness

Aerobic fitness, or cardiorespiratory fitness, is the ability of the body's cardiovascular and respiratory systems to supply oxygen to working skeletal muscles for energy production during sustained physical activity. Major contributors to aerobic fitness are the amount of blood your heart can pump per beat (stroke volume), maximum heart rate, cardiac output (the product of heart rate and stroke volume), and arteriovenous oxygen difference (difference of oxygen content between arterial and venous blood). As cardiac output and arteriovenous oxygen difference increase, oxygen consumption increases. Hence, oxygen consumption is a great way to measure aerobic fitness.

There is convincing evidence that a moderate and high level of aerobic fitness reduces the risk of cardiovascular disease-related death and death from any causes in both men and women. High aerobic fitness is also linked to favorable insulin sensitivity, cholesterol levels, body composition, blood pressure, and functioning of the autonomic nervous system. A major benefit of aerobic exercise is increased aerobic fitness.

Muscle Fitness

Muscle strength is a measure of muscle fitness and is defined as the maximum amount of force muscle can exert against some form of resistance at a single time. Muscle strength has a protective effect against death from cancer or any causes in middle-aged adults and is a major physical predictor of frailty, reduced bone mineral density, impaired balance, and falls. The best way to improve muscle fitness is strength exercise.

Body Composition

Body composition refers to the percentages of fat and fat-free mass (e.g., water, muscle, and bone) in the body. Both fat and fat-free mass predict the likelihood of dying from any causes. Excess body fat, particularly abdominal fat, is linked to high blood pressure, insulin resistance, and abnormal cholesterol levels, which collectively are known as the metabolic syndrome. Both aerobic and resistance exercise are important for enhancing body composition.

Balance

Balance is loosely defined as the ability to stay upright or in control of the body movement and can be classified as static and dynamic balance. Static balance maintains equilibrium while being stationary. Dynamic balance maintains equilibrium while in motion.

Poor balance is linked to a high risk of falls. Balance can be improved the most through balance exercise, but aerobic and strength exercises can also increase balance.

Flexibility

Flexibility refers to the ability to move a joint through a complete range of motion. Flexibility is important to perform activities of daily living and prevent debilitating musculoskeletal ailments such as nonspecific low back pain. While flexibility exercise improves flexibility the most, other types of exercise are also important for maintaining or even improving flexibility.

How Does Fitness Change with Age?

Aging is characterized by an inevitable and gradual deterioration of physical abilities and physiological reserves that reduce each type of physical fitness. Aerobic fitness has been shown to decline by 15% to 22% per decade after age 50 in people who did not participate in regular aerobic exercise. This decline means a decreased ability to circulate and use oxygen for energy production.

Sarcopenia (degenerative reduction in muscle mass) is experienced with age, resulting in a corresponding reduction in muscle strength. Muscle strength tends to decline by 30% to 50% between ages 30 and 80. The rate of decline is about 12% to 14% per decade after age 50. In general, people experience greater losses in the lower body strength than in the upper body as a consequence of aging.

Balance depends on the concerted action of both sensory and motor systems. Vision perceives direction and movement. Proprioceptive sensors in the brain, muscles, and joints sense where the body is in space. The vestibular system in the inner ear monitors motion and orients the body. Reaction time determines how quickly a person can respond to a balance change. Muscle strength keeps the body steady. All these systems change with age and affect balance differently among older adults. It has been estimated that one in three old adults falls at least once each year due to balance changes.

How flexibility changes with aging has been less researched. Joint flexibility is estimated to decrease 10% to 40%, depending on the joint.

Change in body composition is another hallmark of aging. Aging typically leads to increased total body fat and decreased lean body mass.

Why Does Fitness Decline with Age?

There are many reasons why physical fitness declines with age. The most common reasons are reduced physical activity, chronic conditions, and disuse.

Reduced Physical Activity

Age-related decline in aerobic fitness likely results from reduced physical activity and exercise. Older adults are generally less active than middle-aged and young adults. Of people aged 50 years old and older, the total amount and intensity of physical activity decrease with age. In relative terms, the amount of moderate-intensity and vigorous-intensity physical activity decreases more than low-intensity physical activity. Total daily physical activity declines by about 2% per year in people aged 70 and older, but the decline accelerates almost twice as fast in those aged 90 and older. Reduced physical fitness makes the performance of activities of daily living more and more difficult and exhausting. Decreased physical activity leads to lower physical fitness, which contributes to more reduction in physical activity, forming a downward spiral.

Chronic Conditions

Diseases, particularly chronic conditions, affect older adults more than young adults. Chronic diseases impact a person's ability to participate in physical activity and exercise. For example, about 50% of older adults have signs of osteoarthritis in their knees. Older women with chronic inflammatory conditions are at higher risk for muscle weakness and physical disability.

Disuse

Disuse happens due to physical inactivity and increasing sedentary behavior (sitting and lying down). Physical inactivity is estimated to be the fourth top-ranked risk factor for death worldwide, leading to about 3.2 million deaths each year. Three-fourths of older adults do not exercise at the recommended level. Older adults also tend to sit more than other age groups, and half describe themselves as sedentary.

However, attributing changes in physical fitness to aging, disease, or disuse alone is an oversimplification of the complex human bodies. Decreasing physical fitness is the result of the interactive effects of aging, disease, and disuse.

Can Fitness Decline Be Prevented?

Although physical fitness decreases with aging, exercise can slow these decreases. The National Institute on Aging of the National Institutes of Health recommends that older adults stay as physically active as they can, because aging, disease, and disuse profoundly affect daily functioning and quality of life. Ample evidence shows that older adults can substantially improve their aerobic fitness, muscle strength, balance, and flexibility through exercise programs well into their 90s.

Age-related decline in physical fitness may even be reversible. For example, older adults who participated in aerobic exercise improved their aerobic fitness 11% to 27%, which sufficiently compensates for the decline due to aging. For the past five years, the American Heart Association has led the effort to establish a national bank to identify the normative values of aerobic fitness for different groups (e.g., age and sex cohorts). Normative values can help benchmark where you are in your aerobic fitness compared with other people like you.

What Are the Health Benefits of Exercise?

Why should you care about exercise if you are not an exercise researcher like us? The top reason is that exercise improves your quality of life. Physical activity and exercise have many well-established health benefits, as summarized below:

- Increased cardiovascular health: Aerobic exercise increases the efficiency and performance of heart muscles and improves the regularity of heart rhythm. It improves both systolic and diastolic blood pressure, blood flow in the heart and throughout the body. Aerobic exercise is an established way to prevent and treat common cardiovascular diseases such as high blood pressure, heart attack (after the acute phase), and peripheral arterial disease.
- Improved physical fitness: Exercise increases aerobic fitness, muscle endurance, balance, and flexibility, which reduces the risk of musculoskeletal disability and falls. Physical activity and exercise reduce fat, particularly in the abdomen; slows the decline in bone mineral density; and increases total body calcium.
- Management of diseases: Exercise regulates cholesterol levels by reducing "bad" low-density and very-low-density lipoprotein cholesterols and triglycerides as well as increasing "good" high-density lipoprotein. It increases

insulin sensitivity, glucose tolerance, and protein synthesis. Exercise is an established non-drug intervention for preventing and treating diabetes, stroke, and high blood pressure. Exercise also prevents some cancers such as breast and colon cancer.

- Psychological well-being: Exercise improve attention span, sleep, mood, sense of accomplishment, perceived well-being, and happiness. It also decreases anxiety, depression, and stress.
- Improved physical function and quality of life: Exercise promotes physical functional performance, functional capacity, and independence. It increases quality of life in older adults.
- Reduced mortality and nursing home placement: Exercise reduces the risk of death in older adults. It also makes them 30% less likely to live in a nursing home.

What Are the Risks of Exercise?

Now that you have heard all of the wonderful benefits of exercise, you should know that exercise does carry some risks. The most serious risk is a cardiac event such as heart attack or cardiac arrest, which can lead to death. Although cardiac events can occur during exercise, in general, moderate-intensity exercise does not cause them in people with healthy hearts. Vigorous-intensity exercise increases the risk of a cardiac event in people with cardiovascular disease, particularly in those who have been previously sedentary. Hence, pre-exercise health screening and aerobic exercise in the right dose at the right time are the best way to lower these risks. You will learn how to minimize exercise risk from our Approach AD S.A.F.E.ly™ pre-exercise health screening and individualized aerobic exercise prescription in Chapter 7.

The most common adverse event from exercise is injuries to the musculoskeletal system. Exercise, particularly when starting or progressing, may cause delayed muscle soreness, pain, and stiffness 24 to 72 hours after exercise. It is believed to be caused by eccentric contractions (contraction while the muscle is lengthening) during exercise, leading to inflammation and small tears to the muscle fibers. It is most notable from strength exercise with a large eccentric component. The best prevention is to slowly increase the exercise dose as outlined by our Approach AD S.A.F.E.ly™ exercise session setup in Chapter 8.

Another risk is that you may not be able to improve your physical fitness. Not everyone benefits from exercise or benefits to the same degree. Staggering variations in fitness gains were first reported in 2001. In studies, some people improved their aerobic fitness by 100%, while others experienced no change or even became less fit, even though they followed the same aerobic exercise program. The "low-sensitivity" to exercise may run in families, suggesting a genetic difference in how human bodies respond to aerobic exercise. Nevertheless, the number of people who experience benefits, such as increased physical fitness, is far greater than the number of people who do not. Even if you fall into the group whose aerobic fitness does not improve, you will still experience the benefits of exercise in many other ways such as improved health, psychological wellbeing, and quality of life which are independent of increased aerobic fitness, as discussed earlier in this chapter.

What Are the Exercise Recommendations?

Exercise recommendations are usually issued by authoritative organizations such as the World Health Organization, the American College of Sports Medicine, the American Heart Association, the National Institute on Aging, and the Centers for Disease Control and

Prevention. They make similar recommendations, but there are minor differences in the terms and doses they use.

Earlier in this chapter, you learned about the four types of exercise and their effects on various aspects of physical fitness. To reap the greatest health benefits, you should participate in all four types of exercise regularly. Whenever you exercise, remember two basic safety principles. First, start low and increase slowly over time to eventually work up to your target intensity and duration. Second, do warm-up and cool-down before and after exercise. These two principles will lower the risk for exercise-related injuries, make exercise enjoyable, and are the foundational principles underlying our Approach AD S.A.F.E.ly™ protocol. Now, let us turn our attention to the current exercise recommendations for older adults.

Aerobic Exercise Recommendations

The American College of Sports Medicine recommends that each week, older adults take part in at least 150 minutes of moderate-intensity aerobic exercise, 75 minutes of vigorous-intensity aerobic exercise, or an equivalent mix of moderate- and vigorous-intensity aerobic exercise.

Some examples of moderate-intensity aerobic exercise include swimming, bicycling, cycling on a stationary cycle, walking briskly on a level surface, and rowing. You can divide your 150 minutes a week in any way that suits your lifestyle (e.g., 30 minutes a session, five days a week; 50 minutes a session, three days a week; 60 minutes a session, two or three days a week; or 10 minutes a time, three times a day, five days a week).

Vigorous-intensity aerobic exercise is appropriate if you have already been regularly engaging in moderate-intensity aerobic exercise. In other words, if you are new to aerobic exercise, vigorous-intensity aerobic exercise is not where you should start. Examples of vigorous-intensity aerobic exercise include climbing stairs or hills, brisk uphill bicycling, swimming laps, cross-country skiing, hiking, and jogging. Older adults are recommended to participate in 75 minutes of vigorous-intensity aerobic exercise weekly. Similar to moderate-intensity aerobic exercise, the weekly dose can be split in ways that suit you such as 15 minutes a session, five days a week or 25 minutes a session, three days a week.

If you are interested in doing a mix of moderate- and vigorous-intensity aerobic exercise weekly, then plan ahead to decide the duration of exercise for each intensity. For example, for a 50-50 split, you can do 50% of the recommended weekly duration for each exercise intensity; that is, 75 minutes of moderate-intensity and about 40 minutes of vigorous-intensity aerobic exercise each week. For a 30-70 split, you could take part in 45 minutes of moderate-intensity aerobic exercise (30% of 150 minutes) and about 50 minutes of vigorous-intensity aerobic exercise (70% of 75 minutes) a week. Again, this mixed exercise regimen is not for people just starting an aerobic exercise routine.

We cannot overemphasize the importance of following the two general safety principles mentioned earlier. To apply the principle, "start low and increase slowly over time," start at a low intensity for a short duration and gradually build your aerobic fitness to reach the recommended aerobic exercise dose over time. During each exercise session, make sure to do warm-up and cool-down before and after exercise.

Let us use our research studies to illustrate how we have used these principles. Our aerobic exercise program is moderate-to-low-vigorous-intensity cycling for 50 minutes a session, three times a week. Our participants started at low-moderate intensity for 20 minutes a session in week one, for a total of 60 minutes a week. If they finished week one without any issues, their exercise intensity was increased by 5% in week two, but their exercise duration remained the same at 20 minutes a session. If they tolerated this increase with no problems in week two, their exercise duration was lengthened by 5 minutes to 25 minutes a session in week three, while exercise intensity was the same as week two. Once our participants got used to this new level, then their exercise intensity was increased by 5% in week four, but the exercise duration stayed the same. This alternate increase in exercise intensity or duration by small amounts were repeated over the following weeks until the participants reached their target exercise doses.

Following the above exercise progression schedule, it usually took about eight weeks for our participants to reach the recommended aerobic exercise dose. Before and after aerobic exercise in each session, our participants did a five-minute warm-up and a five-minute cool-down. This progressive schedule has proven to be very safe and made exercise fun for our participants. Our Approach AD S.A.F.E.ly™ protocol details all aspects of the "how-to" strategies for aerobic exercise that we have tested in our studies in later chapters.

Strength Exercise Recommendations

Strength exercise provides substantial benefits to older adults, including increased muscle, bone, tendon, and ligament strength and joint function to prevent falls. The American College of Sports Medicine recommends that older adults participate in strength exercises on two or more days a week, including eight to 10 exercises that focus on major muscle groups in the legs, hips, abdomen, chest, back, shoulders, and arms.

Start with no weight or small weight (one or two pounds), and gradually add weight over weeks to a challenging amount. Do warm-up range of motion exercise on all joints slowly and stretch after strength exercise. Do not do strength exercises in the same muscle groups two days in a row to allow the muscles to rest between workouts. You can still do other types of exercises, just not strength exercise. If you choose to do strength exercise every day, you should alternate the muscle groups on consecutive days, e.g., strength exercise of upper-body muscles on day one and lower-body muscles on day two. When you exercise a muscle group, take three seconds to lift or push the weight into place, hold the position for one second, and take another three seconds to lower the weight. Do a few repetitions in a row and gradually build up to eight to 12 repetitions in a row over weeks, if you can tolerate.

Balance Exercise Recommendations

Balance exercises are important to prevent falls by improving your ability to stay upright and control body movements and coordination. Some balance exercises build up leg muscles and are similar to strength exercises of the lower body, while others increase stability. You can also add balance modifications to regular lower-body strength exercises. An easy and effective strategy to incorporate balance exercise into your daily routine is to do it "anytime, anywhere," such as shifting your center of gravity to one leg while standing. Once you build stability, consider standing on one leg with the other leg bearing less weight, no weight (barely touching the floor), and then slightly off the floor over weeks.

Flexibility Exercise Recommendations

Older adults are recommended to do stretching exercise at least two days each week for at least 10 minutes each day. Stretch only when your muscles are warmed up (i.e., after an aerobic and strength exercise session). If you have not warmed up your muscles, do some gentle movements or walk slowly for a few minutes and then stretch. If stretching exercise is the only exercise you can do, do it three times a week and gradually build to stretch every day. When you stretch, do shoulder, upper arm, calf, and thigh stretches by holding the stretched position for 10 to 30 seconds, if you can tolerate. Make sure to move slowly into the position instead of jerking into the position. Stretch to the extent of mild discomfort where you can feel the stretch without pain. Aim to reach from 15 to 30 minutes in each stretching session over time.

Table 4.2 providers a summary of the exercise recommendations for older adults. Of importance, even if you do not reach the recommended exercise intensity and duration in any types of exercise recommended above, you will still receive some health benefits. Recent scientific evidence suggests that as little as 10 minutes of moderate-intensity aerobic exercise is beneficial; however, durations shorter than 10 minutes are not long enough to have a therapeutic effect on the heart and lungs. In the long run, you hurt your health far more by not exercising than by exercising.

Table 4.2. Exercise Recommendations for Older Adults

Type	Recommendation
Aerobic exercise	At least 150 minutes of moderate-intensity aerobic exercise; or
	75 minutes of vigorous-intensity aerobic exercise; or
	An equivalent mix of moderate- and vigorous-intensity aerobic exercise
Strength exercise	Two or more days a week, including eight to 10 exercises that focus on major muscle groups in the legs, hips, abdomen, chest, back, shoulders, and arms
Balance exercise	Incorporating into daily routine, and doing it "anytime, anywhere"
Flexibility exercise	At least two days each week for at least 10 minutes each day

What Is New About Exercise?

Research evidence in two particular areas has increased the understanding of the benefits of physical activity and exercise over the past 15 years. First, sedentary behavior, or too much sitting or lying, is increasingly recognized for increasing the risk of chronic diseases, particularly cardiovascular disease and diabetes. Sedentary behavior is found to make up 55% of the waking hours in 20 to 29 years old and 67% in 70 to 79 years old. Sitting is associated with all-cause and cardiovascular death. As a result, light-intensity activity is recommended to reduce sedentary behavior, so people can move more and sit less.

Second, high-intensity interval training or HIIT has emerged as effective on managing chronic diseases in adults. HIIT consists of a few minutes of high-intensity exercise alternating with several minutes of low-intensity exercise. The initial benefits from HIIT have been reported in older adults, but its effects are yet to be established.

Key Messages

- Physical activity and exercise are a vital component of healthy aging. Aerobic, resistance, balance, and flexibility exercises, can be performed individually or as part of an exercise program to promote physical fitness (aerobic fitness, muscle fitness, body composition, balance, and flexibility).
- Physical activity and exercise have many health benefits such as improved quality of life, cardiovascular health, psychological well-being, and physical health.
- Although improved physical fitness is not guaranteed for everyone who exercises, the benefits of exercise far outweigh its risks for most people.
- Two general principles to promote exercise safety are to "start low and increase slowly over time" and "do warm-up and cool-down before and after exercise."
- Each week, older adults are recommended to take part in at least 150 minutes of moderate-intensity aerobic exercise, 75 minutes of vigorous aerobic exercise, or an equivalent mix of

these two; strength exercise at least two days a week; balance exercise "anytime, anywhere;" and stretching exercise when the muscles are warmed up.

- Low-intensity physical activity is also beneficial as it breaks sedentary behavior that is detrimental to health.

The Beginning Scenarios

Now, let us return to the five scenarios at the beginning of this chapter. Can you define the type of exercise in each scenario? My mom does a combination of aerobic and flexibility exercises. The fitness program my colleague and I participated in is strength exercise. Tai chi is a combination of balance and leg strength exercises with a meditation component. Square dancing and the fitness classes my committee member attended to are aerobic exercises.

The essence of these scenarios is that a wide variety of exercise options are available for you choose from based on your preference and fitness level as well as the area of physical fitness you want to improve. As the American College of Sports Medicine adeptly put it in its global initiative, Exercise is Medicine®! If you are not currently exercising, we hope that you are now motivated to reap all the health benefits that exercise has to offer. Chapters 7 and 8 will take you through the steps to start and advance your exercise participation safely over time.

Chapter 5

How Is Exercise Beneficial to People with Alzheimer's Disease?

*I*n 2004, I started my postdoctoral training jointly at the Pennsylvania State University and the University of Pennsylvania on a quest to take my dissertation research to the next level. Particularly, I was interested in these questions: How do I build on the success of my dissertation findings, which showed that older adults with cognitive impairment benefited from rehabilitation services similarly to their peers with intact cognition? Why did rehabilitation work despite the popular belief that people with dementia would not benefit? My mentors, Drs. Ann Kolanowski at the Pennsylvania State University and Neville Strump at the University of Pennsylvania suggested that I go back to the literature. So I did. A couple of months later, I rushed into

Ann's office, waving a scientific article, exclaiming that I had found the answer: aerobic exercise.

———————————◆————————◆———————————

Fast forward to 2012. By then, I had completed four pilot studies to develop an aerobic exercise intervention, cycling on recumbent stationary cycles, and test its feasibility and preliminary effects in older adults with Alzheimer's dementia. These studies allowed me to build an interdisciplinary research team with colleagues from exercise physiology, geriatrics, neuropsychology, and biostatistics. I also learned how to recruit older adults with Alzheimer's dementia, screen them for exercise safety, ensure their adherence to the prescribed cycling dose, and train staff to competently work with the participants and their family caregivers. These studies indicated that six months of aerobic exercise improved aerobic fitness and quality of life, maintained cognition and function, and reduced caregiver burden.

———————————◆————————◆———————————

In 2012, I began to develop my first investigator-initiated grant application to the National Institute on Aging of the National Institutes of Health to do a clinical trial. Our team was short of an expert in magnetic resonance imaging (MRI) because MRI had been too expensive to use in my pilot studies. One name came to my mind, Dr. Clifford Jack, Jr., a guru for brain imaging in aging and Alzheimer's disease (AD). I carefully drafted an email to Dr. Jack to try to convince him to join my team. We spoke over the phone, and he agreed to work with me. I really lucked out, because Dr. Jack already believed in the importance of aerobic exercise. In August 2013, the FIT-AD™ Trial (Full title as "Aerobic Exercise in Alzheimer's Disease: Cognition and Hippocampal Volume Effects") was funded by the National Institute on Aging.

I hope the above snippets give you a glimpse into the exciting and fast-moving field of aerobic exercise research in AD. When I first started, there were very few aerobic exercise studies in people with Alzheimer's dementia. By 2019, more than 10 studies have been published, with positive findings. However, it would be amiss not to point out that the findings are inconsistent because the cognitive effects varied from none to large. Improved function and behavioral and psychological symptoms have also been reported. A few studies found a rippling benefit to family caregivers. While the number of studies in people with Alzheimer's dementia are still limited, the scientific evidence from basic science and human studies of people without Alzheimer's dementia is very large, which together supports the notion that aerobic exercise affects brain health and AD through biologically sound mechanisms.

In this chapter, you will read about my journey to identify, develop, and test aerobic exercise for preventing and treating AD. You will learn some major findings from our studies. Next, you will discover the current knowledge about aerobic exercise's effects on cognition and its mechanisms of action on AD brain changes. Last, you will understand the impact of other types of exercise on AD. As you read, please ask yourself how strong you think the scientific evidence is and how much additional evidence is needed to make aerobic exercise a standard treatment for AD.

Why Did I Believe in Aerobic Exercise?

Remember when I rushed into my mentor's office during my postdoctoral training, claiming aerobic exercise was the answer to why rehabilitation worked for improving function in older adults with cognitive impairment in my dissertation study. My excitement was fueled by observing four themes of evidence from the literature in different disciplines that examined the effects of aerobic exercise on cognition from different angles.

Aerobic Exercise's Role in AD

The first theme arose from studies that linked physical activity with reduced cognitive decline and risk for AD. This literature was described in detail in Chapter 3.

The second theme came from the experimental studies, reporting that aerobic exercise interventions produced modest to moderate cognitive gains in adults with intact cognition. A large volume of experimental studies in this area had been completed to warrant the conduct of meta-analyses. A meta-analysis is a statistical method to pull data from individual studies and re-analyze the collective data to overcome the limitations of individual studies, such as small sample sizes or measurement errors. A classic meta-analysis identified 18 studies and found that moderate-intensity aerobic exercise produced moderate cognitive gains, with the most striking improvement in executive function in people with intact cognition.

The third theme originated from experimental studies in older adults with cognitive impairment and dementia, showing that exercise improved cognition, function, and behavioral and psychological symptoms of dementia. A seminal meta-analysis of 30 studies reported that exercise generated moderate cognitive gains. On average, the exercise interventions lasted 45 minutes a session, 3.6 times per week for 23 weeks. Studies not included in this meta-analysis also reported that exercise reduced wandering, aggression, sleep disorders, days with restricted activities, rates of institutionalization, and hypnotic medication use in people with dementia.

The last theme, which emerged from animal studies, suggested that aerobic exercise favorably affects brain structure and function at the molecular and cellular levels. Aerobic exercise reduced neuroinflammation, oxidative stress, and insulin signaling. Most excitingly, aerobic exercise reduced amyloid deposits in AD-transgenic mouse models that were genetically engineered to have AD hallmark brain changes.

These themes of evidence converged to suggest that exercise, particularly aerobic exercise, might modify AD brain changes and symptoms. Would you agree that it seemed logical to think that aerobic exercise could alter the course of AD?

Missing Pieces in Research

Aerobic exercise has been well established as a standard treatment to prevent and treat diseases such as cardiovascular and metabolic diseases. The four trends of evidence suggested that the old wisdom "what is good for the heart is also good for the brain" might indeed have a scientific grounding. However, among the aerobic exercise studies in people with Alzheimer's dementia, the findings were inconsistent, which was largely explained by the different exercise types and doses, lack of measures for aerobic fitness, and poorly characterized study samples.

The prescribed exercise types included aerobic, strength, balance, and flexibility exercises as well as their combinations. The doses varied greatly from study to study: one to five times a week; 20 to 40 minutes a session; very low to moderate intensity; and five weeks to four years in the program duration. The doses rarely met the weekly 150-minute moderate-intensity recommendation for older adults. Participants' adherence to the target exercise dose varied tremendously from 10% to 90%. For example, one study reported that the participants reached only 17% to 34% of the target minutes of exercise. If an aerobic exercise intervention was not done for the intended dose, would you expect to see any benefits?

Aerobic fitness was rarely measured in the aerobic exercise studies in people with Alzheimer's dementia. As described in Chapter 4, aerobic fitness refers to the body's ability to deliver and use oxygen and typically increases as a result of regular aerobic exercise. To this end, aerobic fitness helps to measure how successfully an aerobic exercise program was delivered. In addition, aerobic exercise studies in adults with intact cognition had linked enhanced aerobic fitness to cognitive gains.

The study samples were often selected based on cognitive impairment or dementia with a lack of well-characterized participants with Alzheimer's dementia. Although all dementias share common clinical symptoms as discussed in Chapter 1, AD brain processes differ from other dementias; hence, selecting participants with Alzheimer's dementia is important but requires substantial clinical and research resources.

A Research Vision

In Alzheimer's dementia, cognition and function progressively decline over eight to 12 years. During the moderate-to-severe stages of Alzheimer's dementia, people tend to be admitted to nursing homes because they can no longer recognize their families and/or their care needs exceed the family's abilities to take care of them at home. Hence, the vision of my research program was to promote cognition, functional independence, and quality life for people affected by AD. In older adults with Alzheimer's dementia, I hope to flatten the declining trajectory in cognition and function as much as possible for as long as possible as illustrated by Figure 5.1. When the trajectory begins to drop, it would be a steeper or faster drop over a shorter period of time. By changing the trajectory this way, people with Alzheimer's dementia would have a longer period of relatively higher function, better quality of life, and delayed nursing home admission. Aerobic exercise was the first intervention I put faith in to alter the declining trajectory of AD.

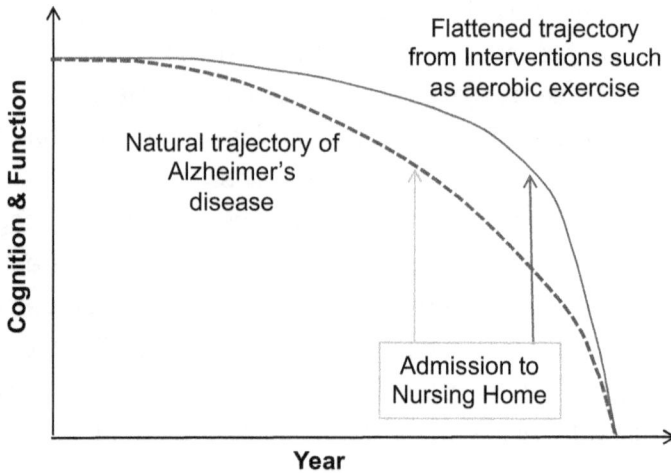

Figure 5.1. Fang Yu's Vision of Research

What Have Your Studies Found?

While we set up the exercise studies to test research ideas, working with the participants and families has been the most gratifying and rewarding aspect of our research. They have been so appreciative of our exercise program, and many have regarded it as the best thing that has happened to them for having AD. In this section, we highlight some results from our studies. If you want to read our published papers, please see the references.

Low Aerobic fitness

One of the ways we measure aerobic fitness is peak oxygen consumption denoted while the participants followed through an exercise testing protocol. The test includes three stages and lasts about eight to 12 minutes. Participants cycle on a recumbent stationary cycle and wear a mouthpiece, which collects the breathed air, and a 12-lead electrocardiogram, which monitors their heart rate and rhythm. During the test, the participants begin to pedal at a speed comfortable to them at about 40 to 60 revolutions per minute. In the last minute of each stage, blood pressure, heart rate, and rating of perceived exertion are recorded. The test ends when the participants cannot maintain the speed, are fatigued, or ask to stop. The breathed air is analyzed to generate peak oxygen consumption. After the test, we monitor participants for six minutes or until their heart rates and blood pressure return to resting levels.

Our studies were one of the first to report peak oxygen consumption from such a test in older adults with Alzheimer's dementia, so there are limited data with which to compare our results. A few other studies have reported peak oxygen consumption from treadmill tests, but comparing peak oxygen consumption from cycling to that on a treadmill is like comparing apple to oranges. However, there is a way to make an apple-to-apple comparison. In healthy, middle-aged adults, peak oxygen consumption obtained from a cycle-based test is typically 10% to 20% lower than that from a treadmill test. By increasing peak oxygen consumption values from our studies by 10% to 20%, we can compare them with those from treadmill tests. Of course, this is a crude comparison.

Our participants showed, on average, a peak oxygen consumption of 1242 ml/min, or 16.9 ml/kg/min. Men had a higher peak oxygen consumption (1383 ml/min, or 17.6 ml/kg/min) than women (1061 ml/min, or 15.9 ml/kg/min). After applying a 10% to 20% increase in peak oxygen consumption, male participants would be expected to have a corresponding peak oxygen consumption of 19.4 to 21.1 ml/kg/min, while female participants would have a peak oxygen consumption of 17.5 to 19.1 ml/kg/min. These adjusted values are very similar to what other researchers have reported from treadmill tests for this population. The gender difference in aerobic fitness is expected. Aerobic fitness in women is typically 20% to 25% lower than that in men because men's hearts are larger than women's, and men have more hemoglobin in their blood and less body fat than women.

When compared with normative peak oxygen consumption from cycle-based tests in healthy older adults 70 to 79 years old, our participants (on average 78 years old) had a lower peak oxygen consumption. The average peak oxygen consumption in healthy older adults ranges from 20.5 to 23.2 ml/kg/min in men and 14.6 to 18.3 ml/kg/min in women, depending on the studies.

Improved Physical Function and Fitness

On average, our participants attended about 74% of the prescribed exercise sessions. Starting with just a couple of miles at the beginning, most participants cycled 10 to 20 miles per exercise session over time. Just to give you a sense of their accomplishment, when we added the total miles a typical participant had cycled in six months, the participant would have biked from Edina, Minnesota to Saskatchewan, Canada, or 860 miles, equivalent to a 14-hour nonstop car trip.

Our participants have shown improved aerobic fitness. We have used several measures to assess aerobic fitness. One measure depicts the lowering of heart rate for the same exercise intensity over time during an exercise test due to improved heart efficiency— exactly what we observed in our participants. Another measure is the increased peak walking speed on the shuttle walk test. After completing the cycling intervention, our participant's peak walking speed had increased.

Stabilized Cognition

Because existing exercise studies lacked a consistent cognitive measure, we selected the Alzheimer's Disease Assessment Scale–Cognition (ADAS-Cog) to measure cognition. The ADAS-Cog has been widely used in AD drug trials, which allows us to benchmark the effects of aerobic exercise on cognition against those of AD drugs. Data from AD drug trials indicate that ADAS-Cog scores naturally increase, on average, 3.14 points over six months (representing worsening cognition) in people with mild to moderate Alzheimer's dementia. In comparison, AD drug studies showed a change in ADAS-Cog scores from a 1.9-point decrease to a 3-point increase over six months. The ADAS-Cog scores in our participants increased only 1.6 points. This means that aerobic exercise has similar cognitive effects as AD drugs.

About 65% of our participants experienced either an improvement or no change in their ADAS-Cog scores. Improved aerobic fitness appears to explain the favorable cognitive change in our participants because the six-month change in aerobic fitness was moderately correlated with the six-month change in cognition.

Reduced Caregiver Burden

The cycling intervention had a ripple effect on family caregivers. We observed a significant reduction in caregiver stress over time, which we anticipated, due to the built-in respite for family caregivers. On the days they exercised, the participants were with our staff for roughly two hours (one hour on the road and one hour in exercise), giving caregivers a six-hour respite per week. However, participants and families reported other benefits in quality of life that we did not to capture with our instruments.

Here are some quotes from our participants: "Sometimes when you have Alzheimer's, you feel kind of alone. [When you exercise with other people], then you do not feel so odd." "If you want to maintain and take care of yourself and not have your family put you away, you would better exercise." "My days will not be the same [without exercise]." "Never wanted to miss a session." "Really enjoyed the program." "Really looked forward to future sessions."

"Gave value to life." "Nothing bad to say [about the exercise program]." "Good relationships with other participants."

Feedback from family caregivers has been overwhelmingly positive: "Dignified way to accept help, in terms of accepting rides and creating daily and weekly structure." "The study was nothing but positive." "Very nice for me! Respite care." "Opened up the talk about AD at home." "HUGE for us as caregivers!" "Took a bad thing and turned it good." "Amazing opportunity to exercise and socialize." "Cream of the crop!!" "Got the ball rolling for participation in other activities." "Everyone was patient and respectful." "[Mom] thought she had achieved something, and it made her more positive." "I think one thing it made me feel good is that something was being done that was positive because I get tired of going to the doctor and having him say, 'Well, there is not much we can do for Alzheimer's.'"

What Is the Collective Evidence?

Since my journey into aerobic exercise for AD in 2004, the number of experimental studies of aerobic exercise in AD has been growing around the globe, showing that aerobic exercise produces mild to large effects on cognitive, functional, behavioral and psychological symptoms in all phases of AD. However, the findings have been mixed, with some studies finding no effects and others reporting large effects. The differences in findings may be attributable to variability in study designs and study samples.

Quite a number of meta-analyses have also been performed on aerobic exercise's effect on cognition, reporting no, modest, moderate, or large effects. The inconsistent findings are explained by the exercise types (analyzing all exercise types together or just aerobic exercise), statistical methods used for the analyses, AD phases targeted, and specific studies included in the analysis. A 2018 meta-analysis in the *Journal of the American Geriatrics*

Society identified 19 experimental studies published from 2002 to 2015: eight studies in people at risk for Alzheimer's dementia and 11 in people with Alzheimer's dementia. Sixty-five percent of the studies used primarily aerobic exercise interventions and 35% used a combined intervention (aerobic plus strength exercises). Overall, exercise showed a modest favorable effect on cognition, but aerobic exercise had a moderate effect on cognition in people with Alzheimer's dementia. Greater exercise adherence was associated with greater cognitive improvement. The aerobic exercise program was, on average, moderate intensity for 45 minutes per session, 3.4 days per week for 137 minutes per week.

Aerobic exercise's effect on cognition in Alzheimer's dementia may result from improved aerobic fitness. Enhanced aerobic fitness has been linked to improved brain volume, functional connectivity, and cognition in adults with intact cognition. A recent clinical trial did not find cognitive benefits from a six-month aerobic exercise program in people with Alzheimer's dementia but did find that enhanced aerobic fitness was associated with less cognitive decline over time.

How Does Exercise Alter Brain Reserve?

Aerobic exercise induces structural changes in the brain by increasing gray matter volumes in the frontal, parietal, and temporal lobes. Six to 12 months of aerobic exercise can increase hippocampal volume up to 2%. Aerobic exercise also improves blood flow to the brain, which increases the brain's oxygen and glucose uptake and use. These positive changes likely underlie aerobic exercise's effect on improved functional connectivity among different regions of the brain.

On the molecular level, aerobic exercise increases the formation of new neurons and synapses and improves the production and function of neurotransmitters. A key regulator of brain reserve is the brain-derived neurotrophic factor (BDNF). BDNF is a protein that helps produce new brain cells, protect brain cells from damage, repair damaged cells, and promote the function of brain cells. It also plays an important role in helping synapses adapt to changing conditions, particularly in the hippocampi where memory is made. Aerobic exercise has long been known to increase the production and function of BDNF. In animal studies, BDNF was found to mediate the effects of aerobic exercise on the formation of new neurons and increase hippocampal volume. In humans, higher BDNF levels have been associated with better cognition and slower cognitive decline. Aerobic exercise is well-known to increase blood BDNF levels in animals and humans.

Aerobic exercise also induces other growth factors similar to BDNF, such as insulin-like growth factor 1 and vascular endothelial growth factor. Insulin-like growth factor 1 helps newly generated neurons survive and improves memory, while vascular endothelial growth factor regulates neural growth. These proteins also enhance the generation of blood vessels and increase capillary density and branching in the brain, which improves the exchange of oxygen and nutrients and helps the brain rid itself of waste. Levels of BDNF, insulin-like growth factor 1, and vascular endothelial growth factor are all lower than normal in AD.

How Does Aerobic Exercise Modify AD?

The ways aerobic exercise works in many diseases that occur outside the brain have already been studied extensively. In the past two decades, a very large literature has accumulated on how aerobic exercise affects AD hallmark and non-hallmark brain changes in basic science and through AD biomarkers. AD-transgenic animal models, which carry AD genes taken from humans and transferred to their genetic makeup, have been widely used to uncover the mechanisms of action of aerobic exercise in AD. AD biomarkers described in Chapter 2 allow such mechanistic studies in living humans.

Amyloid Plaques

The large number of studies using AD-transgenic animal models generally support that aerobic exercise modifies AD hallmark brain changes, but show varying strengths of aerobic exercise's effects. The varying strengths are due to the differences in the experimental methods used, such as the type and age of AD-transgenic animal models; the timing and dose of the aerobic exercise interventions; and the specific methods used to analyze brain changes.

Aerobic exercise is found to change the processing of amyloid precursor protein to amyloid-beta (Aβ) and the degradation and clearance of Aβ. Aerobic exercise suppresses the activity of β-site APP cleaving enzyme 1 and increases the activities of α- and γ-secretases, leading to the formation of more nontoxic amyloid segments and fewer toxic Aβ segments. Aerobic exercise increases the production and function of enzymes that degrade and remove Aβ from the brain through the blood-brain barrier. Aerobic exercise also reduces soluble Aβ oligomers, which are increasingly recognized for their roles in AD brain changes.

A few observational studies have correlated physical activity with reduced Aβ in the cerebrospinal fluid or blood, but the results have been mixed. Aerobic exercise has been associated with reduced Aβ levels in the brain in people without dementia but not in people with mild cognitive impairment or mild Alzheimer's dementia. While experimental studies are greatly needed to establish the effects of aerobic exercise on Aβ biomarkers in AD, there is a cost issue. Imaging and cerebrospinal fluid biomarkers of Aβ are expensive. If the meaningful change in Aβ is relatively small, a large number of participants must be enrolled in order to detect the change, which further increases the cost of running aerobic exercise studies.

Neurofibrillary Tangles

Aerobic exercise was shown to reduce tau hyperphosphorylation in the hippocampus and cortex of AD-transgenic animal models. The findings are mixed, which is again largely explained by the type and age of the animals and the timing and dose of the aerobic exercise intervention. Emerging research suggests that aerobic exercise increases the abundance and activity of several tau-regulating enzymes and genes that decrease tau hyperphosphorylation and help expel abnormal tau. Few studies have examined the effects of aerobic exercise on abnormal tau in humans.

Neurodegeneration

In the past, scientists thought that humans were born with a set number of neurons for life. Today, it is recognized that neurons can regrow and that newly produced neurons can be integrated into the existing neural networks to perform different functions. Wheel running produced favorable brain changes in mice, such as an enlarged hippocampus, and increased expression of genes that promote the growth and function of neurons and capillaries.

In human studies, aerobic exercise has been shown to reduce brain tissue loss and increase gray matter volume and blood flow to many areas of the brain. These changes have been seen in older adults with intact cognition and in those with preclinical AD.

Oxidative Stress

In the short term, exercise stresses the body by increasing the metabolic demand that causes the production of free radicals, mostly from skeletal muscles. For individuals with no exercise training, the level of oxidative stress biomarkers increases considerably after exercise. In contrast, exercise over time or chronic exercise helps the body adapt to oxidative stress. Regular exercisers show little change in oxidative stress biomarkers before and after exercise. Regular exercise also boosts the antioxidant defense systems to reduce oxidative stress.

Scientists have seen similar effects of exercise on animal brains. Regular aerobic exercise improves mitochondria function, reduces the damage of oxidative stress to neurons, and increases the brain's antioxidant defense. In studies of AD-transgenic mice, aerobic exercise normalized oxidative stress levels in the brain caused by AD and reduced oxidative damage to fats and DNA, particularly in the hippocampi. Few studies have examined how aerobic exercise affects oxidative stress in the brain of living humans.

Insulin Resistance

Aerobic exercise helps the body use glucose by moving it from the blood to the muscles, which is why aerobic exercise is used as a treatment for pre-diabetes and diabetes. Aerobic exercise has been found to improve insulin signaling in the brain. In a study of healthy adults, 12 weeks of aerobic exercise significantly improved glucose use in the areas of the brain often affected by AD.

Neuroinflammation

Both occasional and regular exercise reduces inflammation throughout the body. The anti-inflammatory effect from one exercise session is immediate but short-lived, while regular exercise has a lasting effect. A 16-week aerobic exercise program significantly reduced pro-inflammatory cytokines such as tumor necrosis factor-α in the blood in people with mild cognitive impairment.

Cardiovascular Conditions and Risk Factors

Aerobic exercise improves cardiovascular function in several ways. The brain gets its energy from oxygen and glucose in the blood. Hence, the brain critically depends on the cardiovascular system to deliver oxygen and glucose, which could be the reason why enhanced aerobic fitness has been linked to favorable cognitive changes.

Aerobic exercise is a well-established, first-line treatment for several cardiovascular conditions and risk factors that are shared by cerebrovascular disease and AD, such as high blood pressure, high cholesterol, diabetes, and obesity. Furthermore, aerobic exercise temporarily increases blood flow to the brain, which, however, quickly returns to normal afterward. Regular exercise does not seem to affect blood flow to the brain, but lifelong exercise may stem the age-associated reduction in blood flow to the brain by about 10 years. Last, aerobic exercise may also protect the brain by increasing the elasticity and function of blood vessel walls and reducing damage to the blood-brain barrier, which creates a favorable environment for neurons.

Apolipoprotein E

In Chapter 3, you learned that carriers of the apolipoprotein E (*APOE*) gene allele 4 (ε4) are at an increased risk for AD. AD-transgenic ε4 mice indeed show poorer memory and learning than ε3 mice. However, aerobic exercise was found to restore cognitive performance in ε4 mice to the level of ε3 mice. More interestingly, aerobic exercise generated greater cognitive benefits in ε4 carriers than non-carriers in humans. These findings suggest that ε4 carriers who are more susceptible to cognitive decline may benefit more from aerobic exercise.

How Do Other Exercises Affect Cognition?

While the focus of our book is on aerobic exercise, it would be amiss if we did not mention the growing interest in the cognitive effects of other types of exercise. Strength exercise generated no to moderate cognitive gains in healthy adults older than 50 and people with mild cognitive impairment, most notably in executive function. In these studies, the exercise took place two or three times a week, involved progressively increased intensity, and lasted longer than six months. Strength exercise is thought to increase growth factors such as BDNF, insulin-like growth factor 1 and vascular endothelial growth factor, and reduce oxidative stress and neuroinflammation to produce cognitive benefits.

No to large cognitive gains have also been observed from yoga and Tai-Chi in people with mild cognitive impairment and dementia. Both yoga and Tai-Chi challenge flexibility and balance and focus on breathing, mindfulness, and meditation. Their cognitive benefits may be achieved through improved sleep, mood, and neural connectivity, as well as reduced stress.

Nonetheless, the number of studies on the effects of resistance, balance, and flexibility exercises on cognition in people with mild cognitive impairment or Alzheimer's dementia has been limited. The exercise doses vary considerably from study to study, which partially explains the inconsistent findings.

Key Messages

- Our work on aerobic exercise in AD was grounded in the scientific evidence showing that physical activity was linked to a reduced risk for AD; aerobic exercise produced cognitive gains in adults with intact cognition, cognitive impairment, and dementia; and aerobic exercise modifies AD brain changes.

- We aimed to develop and test non-drug interventions such as aerobic exercise to ultimately improve functional independence and quality of life for people with Alzheimer's dementia and their family caregivers.
- Since 2005, our interdisciplinary research team has been conducting experimental studies to test the effects of a six-month moderate-to-vigorous intensity cycling intervention on AD symptoms and brain changes. Results from our studies show that older adults with Alzheimer's dementia had low aerobic fitness; six-month cycling improved physical function and fitness, maintained cognition, and reduced caregiver burden; and enhanced aerobic fitness was correlated with less cognitive decline.
- Albeit being mixed, the current scientific evidence, in general, supports the beneficial effects of aerobic exercise on Alzheimer's symptoms.
- A large literature indicates that aerobic exercise boosts brain and cognitive reserve and affects both AD hallmark and non-hallmark brain changes.
- Emerging evidence suggests that resistance, balance, and flexibility exercises may produce cognitive benefits through biologically sound pathways.

The Beginning Scenarios

Now, let us reflect on the three scenarios at the beginning of this chapter. Are you convinced of the role of aerobic exercise in treating AD? How strongly do you feel about the evidence to recommend aerobic exercise as a routine treatment for AD? What do you suggest that we should do next to advance the science? To us, the current evidence on aerobic exercise as a therapeutic intervention for Alzheimer's dementia, albeit mixed, is voluminous and favorable.

The Alzheimer's Rx: Aerobic Exercise

Even if its effects on cognition are not always supported, aerobic exercise improves functional, behavioral, and psychological symptoms as well as quality of life. Other experts think so too because the World Health Organization recommends engaging in moderate-intensity aerobic exercise at least 150 minutes per week, vigorous-intensity aerobic exercise for 75 minutes per week, or a combination of the two, plus muscle-strengthening training two or more days a week to promote brain health and prevent AD.

Chapter 6

How Can Person-Centered Care Be Used to Ensure Exercise Safety?

Sarah, our exercise specialist, noticed that some research participants were not increasing their resistance or speed over time on the recumbent stationary cycle. We wanted participants to increase their exertion by alternately increasing resistance and speed to reach their individualized target levels. However, some participants slowed down when the resistance was increased because they forgot the speed goal, although they were fully capable of meeting it. Verbal reminders worked inconsistently, so Sarah started to post sticky notes with the target speed next to the speed display on the *cycle. The participants really liked the note because it kept them on speed.*

One day, Kaitlan, a nursing student, was driving a research participant named Mary home after her exercise session. Kaitlan stopped at a stop sign and saw two pedestrians on the other side of the street talking. Because they did not indicate an intention to cross the street, Kaitlan drove on but was pulled over by police. She was cited for not yielding to the pedestrians. Mary appeared very calm and did not say anything while the officer issued Kaitlan a ticket. Kaitlan talked with Mary about the incident after the police left to make sure Mary was ok. Later, Kaitlan contested her ticket in court and had it dismissed. A few months later, Kaitlan was driving Mary home again. Mary asked her what happened to her ticket. Kaitlan was out of words that Mary remembered.

After meeting Anne, a research participant, at the gym for an exercise session, Kaitlin, our exercise specialist and co-author of this book, walked with her towards the cycles. In the split second when Kaitlin craned her neck to see which cycle was available, Anne disappeared. Kaitlin alerted the front desk and police right away. People searched the gym and its neighborhood. Surveillance video revealed that Anne had not left the gym. Anne's family was called and arrived at the gym. An hour later, Anne emerged walking out of another exercise room. She had followed a group of exercisers to that room. Anne said that she knew she was in the wrong place but did not know what to do, so she stayed there, just out of the line of sight from the door when Kaitlin peeked inside searching for her.

To ensure participant safety, Dereck, co-author of this book, and I visited the exercise sessions randomly to see how well our exercise specialists were doing their job. We chatted with the participants but mostly stayed out of sight. Based on our observations, we provided additional training and feedback to the exercise specialists. In one of the sessions, three participants were cycling together. Once settled into a cycling level, one participant, Margaret, pulled out a notebook and started to draw. By the time she was done cycling, she had completed a beautiful sketch of a woman exercising on an elliptical machine. Guess what Margaret's exercise intensity was? Right within her target level!

We hope these scenarios give you a hint into the importance of person-centered care to helping people affected by AD exercise safely. Person-centered care is the cornerstone for ensuring the well-being of this population. When accidents do occur, drawing on person-centered care makes a bad situation better.

In this chapter, you will learn about person-centered care, which has been used as the foundation to design our individualized exercise program for people affected by AD to ensure exercise safety and enjoyment. Then, you will be introduced to our Approach AD S.A.F.E.ly™ protocol which we have developed, tested, and fine-tuned over 15 years of aerobic exercise research. Next, you will become familiar with how AD affects communication. Last, you will apply our SLO-BUTS Tool to ensure effective communication and interaction with people affected by AD. This chapter addresses you as an exercise provider or a family caregiver, and an individual affected by AD as the person.

What Is Person-Centered Care?

Person-centered care represents a paradigm shift in health care and calls for considering the patients such as people with Alzheimer's dementia as equal partners in their care. In the past, health care providers gathered information from proxies such as family members under the assumption that people affected by AD, especially those with Alzheimer's dementia, could not give reliable information or are not capable of participating in their own care. However, extensive evidence now shows that people with Alzheimer's dementia adjust their identities and construct new dimensions in their identities—even in the final stage of Alzheimer's dementia.

Person-centered care is also called "patient-centered" or "client-centered" care. There is no single definition for it. In our exercise studies, we defined person-centered care as individualized and coordinated care given within a person's context, which supports personhood with compassion and respect for dignity.

In essence, person-centered care regards people who use health care services as equal partners in planning, developing, delivering, and monitoring health care to ensure that the care meets their unique needs. In person-centered care, each person's preferences, values, and family and social contexts (e.g., community, workplace, culture) are considered. The person is made the center of decision-making and recognized as the expert in his or her life and health. Person-centered care also means offering personalized care, support, or treatment.

How Can I Personalize Care in AD?

Promoting Personhood

Personhood encompasses personal worth (valuable to others), agency (able to make things happen in the world), social confidence (reaching out to others), and hope (sense of safety and wellness despite what may happen). People with mild cognitive impairment and Alzheimer's dementia are constantly struggling to maintain and make sense of their personhood by reconciling who they were before AD, who they are currently, and who they will become when their AD worsens.

Increasing a sense of contentment, social connectedness, self-reliance, and personal growth helps promote personhood in people with Alzheimer's dementia. Like everyone else, people affected by AD experience mixed emotions such as sadness and an overall sense of contentment with their lives. The sense of contentment can overshadow the negative emotions, but it depends on how well they accept their cognitive impairment and adjust their life expectations. It also depends on how well family and friends adjust their expectations.

Social connectedness remains very important to people affected by AD. Being connected to family, nature, a larger community, or a social group increases the sense of connectedness.

People affected by AD have rich life experiences and express confidence in coping with both prosperity and adversity and making the best out of their remaining life. Maintaining this sense of self-reliance helps promote their sense of independence in light of their feelings of insecurity and limitations in their daily activities.

Continued personal growth is a source of enjoyment that brings meaning and satisfaction to people affected by AD. This may mean participating in different leisure activities, exploring new places, and visiting foreign countries.

Three Steps

Applying person-centered care in AD begins with assessment. Assessment means gathering the essential information to understand the person and his or her family and social contexts; AD symptoms and their impacts; and useful strategies for addressing AD symptoms. Another aspect of assessment is to screen for exercise safety and recognize the barriers and facilitators to exercise, which will be detailed in Chapter 7.

Next, meet the person affected by AD where he or she is. Work with the person to set attainable goals and create a plan. In other words, interact with the person in a way that capitalizes on his or her abilities rather than limitations.

Last, adjust care as the person and his or her family and social contexts change. In Chapter 1, we described AD as a biological continuum with three phases (preclinical AD, mild cognitive impairment due to AD, and Alzheimer's dementia) and Alzheimer's dementia moving through mild, moderate, and severe stages. As AD brain changes accumulate over time, the symptom clusters and their impacts on a person also change; hence, strategies that worked yesterday might not work today or in the future. Figure 6.1 illustrates the circular processes of the three steps.

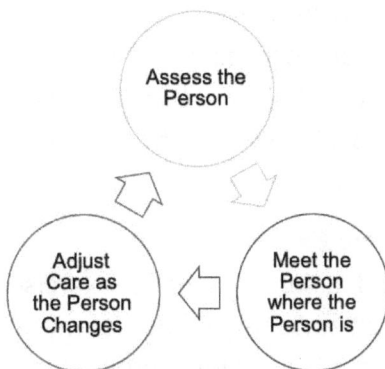

Figure 6.1. Application of Person-Centered Care

How Was the Approach AD S.A.F.E.ly™ Protocol Developed?

When I first began exercise research in older adults with Alzheimer's dementia, there was a lack of existing aerobic exercise programs and guidelines for this population. It was unclear if older adults with Alzheimer's dementia could feasibly and safely participate in aerobic exercise given their impaired cognition, communication, judgment, physical function, and behavioral and psychological symptoms of dementia. It was also unclear if they could exercise to a level that would enhance their aerobic fitness. Neither was there an established approach for screening for exercise safety and monitoring exercise responses that were specifically suitable for this population. Using person-centered care and exercise safety as the founding principles, I have led my team to develop and test the following processes through multiple studies.

Screening for Exercise Safety

We first screened older adults with Alzheimer's dementia for exercise safety over the phone to identify any medical conditions that could make exercise risky. Then the potential participants and their families were invited to an in-person interview in which we obtained the participants' health history. Afterward, we contacted the participants' health care providers to verify that exercise is safe from the providers' perspectives. Last, the participants took part in an exercise test where their heart rhythm was monitored with an electrocardiogram to identify any abnormal and unknown heart conditions.

Selecting an Aerobic Exercise Mode

After I compared different aerobic exercise options, I chose cycling on recumbent stationary cycles for my studies. Cycling was the winner because of its safety features of being recumbent, stationary, and easy on the joints. Imagine if a person with Alzheimer's dementia became confused when cycling, forgot what he or she was doing or simply wanted to stop, he or she would still be sitting with a back support, just like sitting in a chair. The chance of falling off the cycle is much lower than that from a treadmill or non-recumbent exercise machines. Cycling motions are very intuitive and do not require prior experience or skill. Recumbent cycles are not weight-bearing, which is easy on the joints because knee and hip arthritis are very common in older adults. The decision to go with cycling has rewarded us handsomely over the past 15 years because no participants have experienced cycle-related adverse events, although we have seen a wide variety of AD symptoms that might have affected exercise safety if we had used other exercise equipment.

Determining the Exercise Prescription

We designed the cycling intervention based on the recommended moderate-intensity aerobic exercise for 150 minutes per week for older adults. Our cycling prescription was standardized as supervised, 50 minutes a session, three times a week for six months. Standardization is paramount in experimental studies to minimize spurious results, so participants exercise in a systematic way that is comparable and consistent no matter who the exercise specialists and participants are. Standardization also allows the real-world adoption of the aerobic exercise intervention by the public and the replication of studies by other researchers.

Exercising three times a week ensured that the amounts of travel and exercise were not too burdensome to the participants. Spacing exercise sessions out also allowed the participants to recover between sessions. Six months were chosen as the program duration because studies suggested that six months were sufficient to produce cognitive gains in adults with intact cognition and to make permanent behavioral changes such as making exercise part of a person's routine.

Individualizing Exercise Intensity

Because each person has his or her own level of exercise capacity, an exercise program needs to be individualized. In our exercise studies, we individualized moderate intensity for each participant, while the cycling frequency, session duration, and overall program duration were the same for all participants.

Of the different methods for determining moderate intensity, we have found the combined heart rate reserve and rating of perceived exertion most useful for older adults with Alzheimer's dementia. Heart rate reserve was objectively determined from aerobic fitness tests, while the rating of perceived exertion relied on a participant's own perception of how hard she or he was exercising. Methods for determining heart rate reserve and using the rating of perceived exertion scale will be detailed later in Chapters 7 & 8. Our studies started with testing moderate-intensity cycling and progressed to include low-vigorous intensity later. The moderate-to-low-vigorous intensity was individualized as 65% to 75% of heart rate reserve or a rating of 10 to 14 on the rating of perceived exertion scale.

Progressing to the Target Dose

In Chapter 4, we advised that older adults start low and increase slowly over time to work up to the target intensity and duration and do a warm-up and cool-down before and after exercise at the target intensity. While our cycling prescription was 65% to 75% of heart rate reserve or a rating of 10 to 14 on the rating of perceived exertion scale for 50 minutes, three times a week, our participants did not get to this level until about week eight. They started at 40% to 55% heart rate reserve or a rating of perceived exertion of seven for 15 to 20 minutes a session in the first week. If they did well, the intensity was increased by 5% of heart rate reserve or one level up on the rating of perceived exertion scale while keeping the exercise duration the same. The following week, the intensity was kept the same but the participants cycled five minutes longer a session. This alternate increase in intensity and duration continued until the participants reached 65% to 75% of heart rate reserve for 50 minutes a session.

The gradual progression to the target exercise dose was also built into each exercise session. In an exercise session, the participants did a warm-up that involved pedaling slowly at a low resistance. The resistance and pedaling speed were alternately increased over five minutes of warm-up to get the participants' heart rates or ratings of perceived exertion to the target level for a session. Once they reached the target intensity of that session, they maintained their resistance and speed for the rest of the session. Afterward, the participants did cool-down by cycling at a speed and resistance that were alternately reduced over five minutes.

Monitoring Exercise Safety

In our studies, our exercise specialists were fully trained in working with people who have Alzheimer's dementia. Each exercise specialist supervised up to three participants a session. The exercise specialists monitored the participants' heart rates using wireless Polar™ heart rate monitors, rating of perceived exertion, talk test (ability to speak a sentence without losing their breath), and any signs and symptoms of overexertion such as overly elevated blood pressure, nausea, and severe shortness of breath every five minutes.

Coordinating Exercise

Our exercise specialists worked with the participants and their family caregivers and primary care providers to coordinate the exercise sessions and care to ensure ongoing exercise safety. The exercise sessions were flexible and met the needs of each participant. To promote personhood, our exercise specialists were trained to demonstrate compassion and respect for people with Alzheimer's dementia. Many of our research participants considered our staff their friends or adopted family members.

The person-centered care approach has worked really well for our exercise intervention. Over the past 15 years, more than 140 older adults with Alzheimer's dementia with an average age of 78 years had participated in our cycling intervention. They attended about 74%–86% of the planned exercise sessions on average, which are remarkable even when compared to the exercise adherence rates among older adults without Alzheimer's dementia. There were some incidents during exercise testing or regular exercise sessions. After completing an exercise test, a participant got dizzy which likely resulted from dehydration. One participant complained of chest discomfort while cycling, but that turned out to be gastric reflux. Our exercise specialist noticed an episode of abnormal heart rhythm in another participant who had no symptoms at all; this condition seemed to be the result of another long-existing disease but had not been picked up before because of its sporadic nature. We worked with the participants' primary care providers and cardiologists on these incidents to ensure ongoing exercise safety for the participants.

Branding the Approach AD S.A.F.E.ly™

After 15 years of developing, testing, and fine-tuning our aerobic exercise program, our brand, the Approach AD S.A.F.E.ly™, was finally born. It originated from the very first phase of aerobic exercise participation: pre-exercise health screening. AD stands for Alzheimer's Disease and S.A.F.E.ly stands for 1) Screen your conditions, 2) Assess exercise readiness, 3) Follow medical evaluation, if needed, and 4) Evaluate fall risk and aerobic fitness.

Although originated from pre-exercise health screening, the Approach AD S.A.F.E.ly™ protocol encompasses more than that. Building on person-centered care, it also includes individualized exercise prescription, exercise session flow, exercise response monitoring during an exercise session, AD symptom management, working with family caregivers and health care providers, and motivating people affected by AD to exercise, which will be discussed in detail in subsequent chapters. We have further developed the Approach AD S.A.F.E.ly™ Instructional Packet that contains the Operations Manual, flow charts, worksheets, and forms for engaging people with Alzheimer's dementia in aerobic exercise.

How Does AD Affect Communication?

A cornerstone of working with people affected by AD is effective communication. When two individuals with intact cognition communicate, the communication process is a two-way street. Both individuals send and receive messages and are responsible for ensuring that they come to a shared understanding. All forms of verbal and nonverbal communication, such as facial expression and body language, are at play.

Since people with preclinical AD have intact cognition (on cognitive tests), their communication is not affected by AD. However, AD begins to affect communication in people with mild cognitive impairment and communication with people with Alzheimer's dementia can be a one-way street. Effective communication with people who have mild cognitive impairment and Alzheimer's dementia starts with an assessment of their levels of awareness about the perceived presence and severity of cognitive impairment and its impact on their abilities to carry out daily activities.

Altered Awareness

People with mild cognitive impairment or Alzheimer's dementia have different awareness about their cognitive impairment and its severity and impact on their ability to carry out daily activities. Assessing the level of awareness helps you meet people where they are by using the appropriate communication methods. It also gives you a sense of how much confidence you can place on how hard they say they have been exercising when you administer the rating of perceived exertion scale to monitor exercise responses.

Similar to AD symptoms, the level of awareness changes over time as AD worsens and can include the following:

- High awareness: People in this group are acutely aware of the extent of their cognitive impairment and its impact on their lives. They are most prone to have reactive depression, grieve their cognitive losses, and worry about the future. The majority of people with mild cognitive impairment fall into this category.
- Partial awareness: Most people with Alzheimer's dementia fall into this category. They have some awareness of their deficits, especially when challenged, but may not dwell on their problems. They "live in the moment."
- No awareness: People with no awareness seem to always forget that they have any limitations due to cognitive impairment. They reject offers of help. It may be very challenging to get them to accept assistance or oversight because they do not perceive the need.

It is important to distinguish these different levels of awareness from denial, a common psychological defense mechanism. However, keep in mind that the boundaries between different levels of awareness are murky. You can get a good grip on a person's level of awareness once you get to know him or her.

Impaired Communication

AD abnormal changes in the brain affect communication and make communication more and more difficult over time. Once people reached the Alzheimer's dementia phase, they cannot consistently convey a message, evaluate whether and to what extent a message is received, or understand a message from others. As a result, communication with people who have Alzheimer's dementia can be a one-way street because the roles of the sender and receiver can no longer be easily switched.

Impaired communication leads to frustration and unmet needs that people with Alzheimer's dementia cannot communicate. The unmet needs in turn trigger behavioral and psychological symptoms of dementia. Hence, you must assume responsibility for making the communication successful, so developing the communication skills to effectively interact with people who have Alzheimer's dementia is an essential and critical skill. You often need to act like a detective to figure out what people with Alzheimer's dementia are trying to tell you.

Factors Affecting Communication

In addition to AD, internal stressors and environmental factors affect communication. Internal stressors include medical factors such as medications, pain, insomnia, fatigue, infection, illness, dehydration, malnutrition, constipation, poor vision, and hearing loss. Emotional stressors such as diminished self-esteem resulting from loss of control, not knowing how to make things happen, fear due to not recognizing people and places, frustration with not being able to communicate normally, lowered frustration and stress tolerance, and perception problems.

People affected by AD, even in the severe stage of Alzheimer's dementia, still perceive cues from the tone of voice and body language. If you appear stressed or hurried, they may focus on that rather than on the content of the conversation. Speaking at a fast pace also undermines communication.

Environmental factors can complicate communication. These factors include an uncomfortable physical space that is too hot, too cold, crowded, or noisy; too much or too little stimulation; a poorly designed physical environment that is hard to navigate because all the doors in the hallways look the same; or a large, open space leading to different rooms or halls.

Communication in Alzheimer's Dementia

Mild cognitive impairment & mild Alzheimer's dementia

Even people with mild cognitive impairment or in the mild stage of Alzheimer's dementia begin to have problems in communication. They have difficulty finding a specific word, often a noun, and describe an item rather than using its name. For example, when trying to say "chair," they might say, "I sit there," "I eat my meal there," or "I read there." They also use generic words that do not have much meaning, such as "thing" or "stuff."

People with mild Alzheimer's dementia also have difficulty understanding abstract thoughts. They might not understand proverbs or figures of speech such as "an apple a day keeps the doctor away." The literal meaning of words and phrases makes more sense to them than the figurative meaning. Memory impairment can cause people with mild Alzheimer's dementia to unknowingly repeat statements or questions and lose track of conversations.

Moderate Alzheimer's Dementia

In moderate Alzheimer's dementia, the inability to communicate effectively becomes more obvious. People with moderate Alzheimer's dementia might forget what they were talking about in the middle of a conversation. They repeatedly ask the same questions or make the same statements. They may use the wrong words or mix up words. Initiating a conversation may be too taxing for them. Their responses to questions become more limited. It becomes more difficult to understand what they are trying to say. As a result, they might refrain from talking much out of worry or embarrassment and avoid social situations.

Severe Alzheimer's Dementia

In severe Alzheimer's dementia, vocabulary is often reduced to a few words or phrases. Comprehension decreases significantly. They might repeat what is said but just a few words or phrases.

Nonverbal communication becomes more important at this point. In the end, people with severe dementia can utter only a few incomprehensible sounds or become mute. Even the ability to follow a simple command may be lost. However, people in this stage still have emotions. Nonverbal means may be the only way they communicate.

How Can I Communicate Effectively?

The Approach AD S.A.F.E.ly™ effective communication calls for assessing the communication ability of people affected by AD and adapting your communication styles to meet them where they are. Any internal and external stressors affecting communication should be addressed. Realistic expectations about their abilities are important so that you can set the right tone and adjust your communication style. Communicate in a familiar and comfortable environment to help the person retain a sense of connection with the surroundings by using visual cues, signs, and labels.

Communication Pitfalls to Avoid

When communicating with people affected by AD, avoid the following communication pitfalls:

- Arguing: Arguing leads to frustration and worsens the situation.
- Giving strict orders: Few people like to be bossed around.
- Being condescending or treating people with Alzheimer's dementia like children: Use the adult tone of voice and respectful words because people with Alzheimer's dementia have rich life experiences.
- Asking questions that require detailed responses: People with Alzheimer's dementia may feel embarrassed, frustrated, depressed, or humiliated if they cannot answer correctly.

- Talking about others in front of people with Alzheimer's dementia: Assume that they can understand everything.
- Asking confrontational questions. Questions like "Do you remember?" are not appropriate. People with Alzheimer's dementia have impaired memory.

The SLO-BUTS Tool

Our Approach AD S.A.F.E.ly™ person-centered communication uses the SLO-BUTS Tool to communicate with people affected by AD. SLO-BUTS, pronounced as "slow buzz," is the acronym of Speak in short sentences; Limit choices; Orient people affected by AD; Break down tasks; Use concrete words; Talk with eye contact and appropriate body language; and Slash distractions.

- Speak in short sentences: Simplify your ideas without talking down to people with Alzheimer's dementia. Speak slowly (one word a second) and in short sentences.
- Limit choices: Avoid open-ended questions. Instead of asking an open-ended question such as "How do you feel today?" Offer specific options such as "Do you have a headache?" or "Did you sleep well last night?"
- Orient people affected by AD: Reintroduce yourself at each visit, and state your name and the purpose of the visit. Ask people with Alzheimer's dementia about their preferred names and use them. People with Alzheimer's dementia often respond to a mood more than spoken words. Smiles and appropriate laughs help set a relaxed tone.
- Break down tasks: Break a task down into a few steps to enhance the feeling of success. Talk through one step at a time.
- Use concrete words: Be specific, and use familiar, concrete words. Convey your message with as few words as possible.

- Talk with eye contact and appropriate body language: Before starting a conversation, make sure that the person knows you are in the room and that you can be easily seen and heard. Establish and maintain eye contact. Use your body posture and language intentionally. Remain calm, interested, and unhurried. Nonverbal communication becomes more important than spoken language as AD progresses.
- Slash distractions: Make the environment free of distractions. Background noises like music, television shows, or loud conversations can be very distracting.

When you cannot understand people affected by AD, take a deep breath, give them your full attention, and listen actively. Focus on a specific word or phrase that seems to have a particular meaning. You may best understand them by being open to hear the emotional tone of the communication, which may prove to be a better means of communication than the spoken words. Most importantly, stay calm and be patient. Ask family members for clues discretely if they are present.

When people affected by AD do not seem to understand you, slow your pace, because you might be talking too fast. Use nonverbal communication such as pointing to a cue or demonstrating the activity being discussed. Consider breaking the task down and show them how to do one step at a time. For example, instead of asking the person to go and sit on a stationary cycle, our exercise specialists would ask the person to walk next to the cycle, then sit on the seat while padding the seat, and then ask them to move a leg over to the other side. If you are in a conversation and feel stuck, you can change the topic and come back to it later.

Key Messages

- Person-centered care treats people affected by AD as equal partners in health care. It is defined as individualized and coordinated care given within a person's context, which supports personhood with compassion and respect for dignity.
- Applying person-centered care is an ongoing, circular process involving three steps: assess the person and his or her context, meet the person where he or she is, and adjust care as the person changes.
- Our Approach AD S.A.F.E.ly™ brand was built on person-centered care and originated from pre-exercise health screening. It also includes effective communication, individualized aerobic exercise prescription, exercise session setup, exercise response monitoring during a session, AD symptom management, motivating people affected by AD to exercise, and working with family and professional caregivers.
- The Approach AD S.A.F.E.ly™ person-centered communication describes the importance of assessing a person's awareness about the presence, severity, and impact of AD on his or her daily life. Most people with mild cognitive impairment have high awareness and most of people with Alzheimer's dementia have partial awareness.
- Cognitive impairment and changing awareness make communication increasingly challenging for people affected by AD. Communication is affected by internal medical and emotional stressors, communication styles of other people, and environmental factors.
- Effective communication further relies on assessing a person's communication ability and adapting your communication to meet the person where he or she is. Avoid communication pitfalls, and use appropriate communication skills.

The Beginning Scenarios

Now let us reflect on the scenarios at the beginning of this chapter. What do you think of the sticky note idea? It seemed simple in retrospect, right? Sarah did not come up with this idea out of the blue. She really got to know the participants and what they could and could not do. In Mary's scenario, Kaitlan had used good communication skills to avoid inflicting emotional distress on Mary. Mary's recall of the traffic ticket was unexpected but in line with an increasing recognition that people with Alzheimer's dementia have lucid episodes when they appear cognitively normal. Lucidity is an area of research funded by the National Institute on Aging. What did you learn about the scenario in which Anne walked away from Kaitlin inside the gym? We changed our procedure and re-trained all staff about how to work with the unanticipated. As for Margaret, Kaitlin really got to know Margaret after talking with her and her caregiver. They realized that Margaret felt cycling was too long and boring and sketching was one of Margaret's hobbies. They together came up with the sketchbook idea. Would it be possible for us to come up with this idea for exercise engagement by ourselves? Most likely not!

Chapter 7

How Do I Start an Aerobic Exercise Program?

Last summer, my brother David was mowing his lawn, and he died of a heart attack on the spot. This has made me really nervous, so I want to start to exercise. I was recently diagnosed with mild cognitive impairment, which is why I contacted you. Unfortunately, your study coordinator said that I am too young to qualify for your study and have to wait a couple of years until I turn 65, but I want to start now. Because of what happened to David, I am hesitant to do so. I do not want to suffer the same fate as him. I know that exercise can be good for my condition, but how do I go about it? I also have an abnormal heart rhythm (atrial fibrillation) and use an inhaler for my asthma." ~Marie, potential research participant

---

"John called after he saw the article about our study in the Star Tribune—Researchers ask: Can exercise slow dementia? He has not been diagnosed with mild cognitive impairment but has noticed changes in his memory. John was never married and lives alone in Saint Paul. He has high cholesterol, diabetes, and obesity. He has never been to a cardiologist and has no signs or symptoms during exercise or at rest. His dad died of a heart attack when he was 72 years old. John used to walk a couple of times a week but not in winter. He plays blackjack with some friends regularly. We have received medical clearance from his primary care provider for proceeding to exercise testing. During exercise testing, our supervising physician noticed ST-segment depression (a sign of narrowed or blocked blood vessels in the heart), so he is trying to find a cardiologist to schedule an appointment." ~Samantha, study coordinator

---

"I was assessing exercise readiness for Frank, a potential client with Alzheimer's dementia. When I asked if he has chest pain at rest or during activity, he pointed to his chest and said 'It burns.' I was immediately concerned and asked him to elaborate. He said that he and his mother have a genetic disorder that increases the risk of heart disease and that he feels burning in his chest every so often. On reviewing his medical history, I saw that he took medications for heartburn. I asked him if he has heartburn, which led to a productive conversation. Frank said that heartburn was indeed the cause of his chest discomfort and that his wife is always on him to watch what he eats and remember to take his heartburn medication." ~Jesse, exercise provider

---

"My client James has Alzheimer's dementia, high blood pressure, and abnormal cholesterol. During my initial evaluation of James' health and medical history, he did not have a diagnosis of heart disease. However, he said that every time he goes for a walk, it feels like he is pulling a wagon, and he feels very tight across his chest and shoulders. I asked him to visit his primary care provider to ensure that he could exercise safely before we do anything else. James heeded my advice and was diagnosed with coronary artery disease. His primary care provider gave me specific instructions on how to modify his exercise program to maximize his safety. James has now been safely exercising under my guidance for the past three months!" ~Michelle, exercise provider

In the preceding testimonials, you read about what is often referred to as the "barriers to exercise," or the things preventing someone from living a healthier lifestyle. You may relate to some of these testimonials or have some of your own. The good news is that it is never too late to start exercising. Although cardiovascular problems during aerobic exercise are relatively rare, they do happen. Therefore, it is important to be proactive and do everything you can to prevent them.

In this chapter, you will get familiar with our Approach AD S.A.F.E.ly™ pre-exercise health screening and individualized aerobic exercise prescription. To keep things simple, this chapter is primarily written to address you as someone who chooses to start an aerobic exercise program on your own or as the client of an exercise provider. Exercise providers refer to personal trainers, aerobics instructors, and health care professionals such as physical, occupational, and recreational therapists, nurses, physicians, and exercise physiologists. Although the Approach AD S.A.F.E.ly™

protocol was developed from aerobic exercise, it is also applicable to other types of exercise.

What Is the S.A.F.E. Tool?

In Chapter 6, we have described that pre-exercise health screening is the first step for ensuring aerobic exercise safety, which gave birth to our Approach AD S.A.F.E.ly™ brand. AD stands for Alzheimer's Disease and S.A.F.E. stands for 1) Screen your conditions, 2) Assess exercise readiness, 3) Follow medical evaluation, if needed, and 4) Evaluate fall risk and aerobic fitness. Steps 1, 2, and 4 are a must. Step 3 can be optional depending on findings from steps 1 and 2.

Screen Your Conditions

Your job, exercise routine, recreational activities, and medical conditions can all affect your ability to exercise. Think about your job, exercise routine, recreational activities, medical conditions, and any signs or symptoms you have had during physical activity and exercise. This will prepare you for the pre-exercise health screening, help you avoid injuries, and establish your baseline exercise level.

Your job, exercise, and recreation

Whether you are working or retired, think about your daily routine. How do you spend your day? Does your job or day involve extended periods of sitting and repetitive movements that cause physical and mental stress? Do you take part in exercise and recreational activities? Focus on the amount, frequency, and intensity of your current physical activity and exercise and the muscles and joints that might be overused or underused on a daily basis. Overall, do you have a sedentary lifestyle with little or no physical activity? Are you meeting the recommended level of exercise described in Chapter 4?

Medical conditions

Cardiovascular, pulmonary, and metabolic diseases could limit the type of exercise you can do; however, aerobic exercise is often a treatment for these diseases. If you have any of the following conditions, it simply means that you should be evaluated by your health care provider before starting a new exercise program or increasing your current level of exercise:

- Cardiovascular diseases involving the narrowing or blockage of blood vessels, such as a coronary artery, peripheral artery, and cerebral artery diseases.
- Nonvascular heart conditions, such as irregular heart rhythm, enlarged heart, and heart failure (heart muscle diseases), or abnormal heart valves.
- Pulmonary disorders which affect levels of oxygen and carbon dioxide in the blood, such as chronic obstructive pulmonary disease, asthma, interstitial restrictive lung disease, and cystic fibrosis.
- Metabolic diseases, which impair energy processing and use, such as diabetes, thyroid disorders, and end-stage kidney or liver diseases.

Even if you have not been diagnosed with these diseases, it is important to identify whether you have had any signs or symptoms of them. The classic symptom of underlying heart disease is chest pain, which may appear differently in men and women. Men commonly have chest pain or discomfort (heaviness, tingling, cramping), nausea, fatigue, shortness of breath, anxiety ("feeling of impending doom"), sweating, dizziness, or pain in the arms, neck, jaw, shoulder, or back. Women may experience these symptoms as well but are more likely to have nausea, stomach pain, shortness of breath, and sharp chest pain (compared with the "pressure" men often describe). In addition to chest pain, other major signs and symptoms include:

- Shortness of breath at rest or mild activity
- Dizziness or fainting
- Leg cramps or tightening while walking
- Racing heart
- Ankle swelling not due to muscle or bone problems
- Heart murmur
- Severe shortness of breath while lying flat or during the night
- Unusual fatigue with usual activity

Complications of diabetes can show up as low and high blood sugar levels. Common signs and symptoms of low blood sugar include shakiness, dizziness, sweating, hunger, anxiety or nervousness, and headache. For high blood sugar, they include increased thirst, blurred vision, frequent urination, fatigue, and problems concentrating. Kidney disease may cause swollen arms and legs, foamy or bloody urine, dry or itchy skin, difficulty sleeping, muscle cramps, and fatigue.

Reasons not to Exercise

If your health care provider has told you that you should not exercise, then exercise is considered unsafe for you. If you do not know whether it is safe for you to exercise, ask your provider.

You should not exercise if you have any of the following conditions:

- Heart attack within two days
- Ongoing, unstable chest pain
- Uncontrolled abnormal heart rhythms that affect heart function
- Active endocarditis (infection of the inner lining of your heart valves and chambers)

- Symptoms of severe narrowing or blockage of the blood vessels in the heart
- Worsening of the signs and symptoms of heart failure
- Pulmonary embolism (a blood clot from the heart to the lungs), pulmonary infarction (death of lung tissue due to blocked blood supply), or deep vein thrombosis (blood clot, usually in the legs)
- Myocarditis (inflammation of the heart muscle) or pericarditis (inflammation of the sac around the heart)
- Aortic dissection (tear in the wall of the artery that carries blood away from the heart)
- Physical disability that makes exercise unsafe

If you have any of these following conditions, ask your health care provider if it is safe for you to exercise:

- Obstructive left main coronary artery stenosis (narrowing or blockage of the arteries that carry blood to the heart)
- Moderate to severe aortic stenosis
- Abnormally rapid heart rhythm with uncontrolled ventricular rates
- Acquired advanced or complete heart block (abnormally slow heart rhythm)
- Hypertrophic obstructive cardiomyopathy (abnormally thick heart muscle that interferes with the heart's ability to pump effectively)
- Recent stroke or transient ischemic attack (brief, stroke-like event)
- Mental impairment that limits the ability to safely cooperate in exercise
- Resting blood pressure with systolic or diastolic blood pressure higher than 200/110 mmHg

- Uncorrected medical conditions, such as significant anemia (low levels of hemoglobin in the blood), important electrolyte (mineral) imbalance such as hypokalemia (low level of potassium in the blood), and hyperthyroidism

Assess Exercise Readiness

Exercise readiness screening helps to figure out whether you will need to see your health care providers before starting an aerobic exercise program if you do not have any of the medical conditions described above. You can use several commonly used screening tools alone or together with your family member or exercise provider, including the Physical Activity Readiness Questionnaire, the ACSM Preparticipation Health Screening Algorithm, and the Exercise Assessment and Screening for You.

Physical Activity Readiness Questionnaire

The Physical Activity Readiness Questionnaire is an easy-to-use tool with seven questions that ask whether you have a heart condition; are on medications; have pain, balance, bone, or joint problems; or any conditions that may prevent you from being physically active. If you answer "no" to all the questions, do not have a family history of cardiovascular disease, and are in good health, you do not necessarily need to get medical clearance to assess your aerobic fitness level and set up an exercise program. If you answer "yes" to one or more questions, you should get a medical clearance before proceeding with the aerobic fitness test or exercise.

The Physical Activity Readiness Questionnaire has limited use for older adults who have one or more chronic conditions because heart conditions and pain, balance, bone, and joint problems are very common in this age group, and their responses to the questions on the Physical Activity Readiness Questionnaire will likely trigger the need for medical clearance unnecessarily. Getting medical clearance before starting an exercise program can be seen as a major barrier to exercise for reasons such as a lack of a regular health care provider and the time and cost of a clinic visit. As a result, other screening tools may be more suitable for older adults and we recommend the following two tools.

2015 ACSM Preparticipation Health Screening Algorithm

ACSM stands for the American College of Sports Medicine. The 2015 ACSM Preparticipation Health Screening Algorithm aims to reduce unnecessary medical clearance to increase exercise participation while ensuring that people who need medical clearance request it. The algorithm states that:

If you do not participate in regular exercise currently:

- If you do not have cardiovascular, kidney, or metabolic disease, medical clearance is not required to participate in moderate-intensity aerobic exercise, which can advance to vigorous-intensity over time.
- If you have cardiovascular, metabolic, or kidney disease or symptoms of them, medical clearance is recommended before participation in a moderate-to-vigorous exercise.

If you currently participate in regular exercise:

- Medical clearance is not required for moderate-intensity aerobic exercise, whether you have cardiovascular, metabolic, or kidney disease or not.
- If you have cardiovascular, metabolic, or kidney disease, it is still considered safe to start a new vigorous-intensity exercise program as long as you had a medical checkup in the past year and your conditions and symptoms have not changed since then. However, if you have any signs or symptoms of cardiovascular, metabolic, or kidney diseases described above, you need to stop exercising and see your health care provider right away.

Exercise Assessment and Screening for You

The Exercise Assessment and Screening for You is a screening tool specifically developed to help older adults identify different types of exercise and physical activity to meet their unique needs and help them choose safe and effective ways to exercise. It has six questions about symptoms during physical activity (chest pain, tightness, or pressure), current symptoms (dizziness and lightheadedness), high blood pressure, musculoskeletal issues (pain, stiffness, or swelling), balance issues, and any concerns about starting an exercise program. Each question answered yes is followed by a decision tree to further elicit the need for medical evaluation and make recommendations about appropriate exercise. Hence, the Exercise Assessment and Screening for You can be very helpful if you are looking to start exercise on your own, particularly if you are thinking of starting different types of exercise programs.

Examples of using the S.A.F.E. Tool

In the following examples, we used all three tools to illustrate that each tool may be useful in different situations.

Donna's story. Donna is a 45-year-old Asian woman. She is an accountant with two teenagers. Both Donna and her husband have worked hard and are mid-level managers in their respective companies. Her parents are in their early 70s and live in the same neighborhood. Her dad was diagnosed with Alzheimer's dementia a couple of years ago. Donna is increasingly stressed by her work (crunching numbers over long hours) and family roles (challenging teenage behaviors at home and caring for her parents). She feels that her memory has been slipping. She missed a couple of deadlines recently and has trouble controlling her temper. Although she used to be physically active, she has not exercised for months.

Donna answered "no" to all questions on the Physical Activity Readiness Questionnaire. She does not participate in regular exercise and has no cardiovascular, pulmonary, or metabolic diseases. Other than a few memory slips and stress, she has no other symptoms and knows how to start an exercise program, so she does not need to complete the 2015 ACSM Preparticipation Health Screening Algorithm and the Exercise Assessment and Screening for You.

Kayla's story. Kayla is a 67-year-old white retiree who lives alone. She worked as a paralegal in a law office for 15 years and spent most of her working hours preparing documents in front of a computer. She has not exercised for many years, but she does all the household chores herself and gardens 20 to 30 minutes daily in the summer. Her favorite activity is watching TV. Her medical history includes Alzheimer's dementia, glaucoma (increased pressure inside the eye), skin cancer, and high blood pressure. Kayla had her last medical visit three months ago. Kayla reports frequent back pain and often feels depressed. She does not want to live in a nursing home and is considering to start an exercise program because it may help her continue to live at home. She has no symptoms during her daily activities.

If we screen Kayla's exercise readiness using the Physical Activity Readiness Questionnaire, her answer to the pain question will be a "yes," which means that she will need medical clearance before starting an exercise program which could deter her motivation to exercise. The 2015 ACSM Preparticipation Health Screening Algorithm will work better. Kayla does not exercise regularly and has no cardiovascular, pulmonary, or metabolic disease or signs or symptoms suggesting otherwise. Therefore, medical clearance is not necessary for Kayla to start moderate-intensity aerobic exercise. The Exercise Assessment and Screening for You has similar suggestions and provided a list of potential exercises for Kayla.

David's story. David is an 82-year-old African American who worked for a medical device company for 40 years before retiring. He traveled a lot for work and was often on his feet when he was on site. He lives at home with his wife. David's last visit to the doctor was six months ago for a urinary tract infection. David's medical history includes mild cognitive impairment, obesity, type 2 diabetes, abnormal cholesterol, macular degeneration (eye disease that can lead to low vision), and coronary artery disease, for which he takes medications. He has no symptoms. He reports being active around the house but has not exercised a day in his life.

On the Physical Activity Readiness Questionnaire, David answered "yes" to at least two questions, which indicates that he needs medical clearance before starting an exercise program. On the 2015 ACSM Preparticipation Health Screening Algorithm, David does not exercise regularly but, unlike Kayla, he has diagnoses of coronary artery and metabolic diseases (diabetes, dyslipidemia, and obesity). The ACSM Preparticipation Health Screening Algorithm and Exercise Assessment and Screening for You both recommend medical clearance.

As the examples illustrate, if you are generally healthy, the Physical Activity Readiness Questionnaire is a quick and easy way to see if you are ready to exercise. The 2015 ACSM Preparticipation Health Screening Algorithm is useful whether you have medical conditions. The Exercise Assessment and Screening for You is best if you are looking to start various exercises.

Follow Medical Evaluation

If medical clearance is required or you have questions about your ability to exercise safely, see your health care provider. In general, if you do not have a history of cardiovascular disease, you can visit your primary care provider for medical evaluation. If you have a history of cardiovascular disease, make an appointment with your cardiologist. If you do not have a cardiologist, then it is a good time to get connected with one. Discuss with your primary care provider or cardiologist the dose of aerobic exercise you plan to engage in (described later in this chapter), so they can better evaluate your exercise readiness and make recommendations.

As part of the medical evaluation, your provider may order a graded exercise test. Graded exercise test traditionally has been used to identify abnormal heart conditions during aerobic exercise, guide aerobic exercise prescription, and gauge treatment responses to aerobic exercise in a clinical or research setting. It typically uses electrocardiography and is performed under the supervision of qualified health care personnel. Graded exercise test requires a progressive increase in the intensity of exercise, or grade, through stages that bring the exerciser to fatigue or cause symptoms. In the United States, the graded exercise test is most often done on a treadmill, but it can also be performed on leg and arm exercise machines.

If you have a graded exercise test as part of your medical evaluation, ask for the documentation of both your resting and peak heart rates during the graded exercise test for your records. If you have these heart rates, you will be able to skip part of step 4 (evaluate aerobic fitness) below and use these heart rates to determine your exercise intensity.

Evaluate Fall Risk and Aerobic Fitness

Your risk for falls needs to be assessed to ensure you can safely take part in an aerobic fitness test and intended aerobic exercise. The main purposes of evaluating aerobic fitness are to examine resting and peak heart rates to individualize exercise intensity and uncover signs or symptoms of hidden cardiovascular disease. Knowing your current state of aerobic fitness will also allow you to compare your fitness to normative values and evaluate the overall effect of your aerobic exercise program over time.

Falls and fear of falling

A fall is when you suddenly find yourself on a lower level without the intention to get there. More than 60% of older adults with Alzheimer's dementia fall each year, and this fall rate is three times higher than those without Alzheimer's dementia. Fear of falling, or being afraid you are going to fall, actually increases the risk for falls. People who fell before are more likely to fall again.

You can use a fall questionnaire to assess your risk for falls on your own such as the Fall Efficacy Scale. This scale asks you to rate your level of confidence on a 1–10 scale when you do 10 different activities such as taking a bath or shower, reaching into cabinets and closets, etc. Your total score ranges from 10 (very confident) to 100 (not confident at all). If you score above 70, then you have a fear of falling.

You can also ask your exercise provider to objectively assess your fall risk using the Timed Up and Go test. The test requires a stopwatch, a standard armchair, and a line 3-foot away on the floor. Your exercise provider will instruct you to "stand up from the chair, walk to the line on the floor at normal pace, turn, walk back to the chair at a normal pace, and sit down again." Your exercise provider will record the time it takes you to complete the test with a stopwatch. If it takes you 12 seconds or more to complete the Timed Up and Go test, then you are at risk for falls. During the test, your exercise provider can also observe your postural stability, gait, stride, and sway. In particular, losing balance, having short strides, having a slow, tentative pace with little or no arm swing, steading self on walls, being unable to use the assistive device properly, shuffling, and requiring multiple small steps to make a turn suggest possible medical conditions that require medical evaluation.

When you have a fear of falling or are at risk for falls, you will need to use fall-prevention strategies. Make sure you wear proper footwear that fit snugly, the environment is well lit, tripping hazards such as a basket in the walkway are removed, and assistive devices such as handrails are used.

Graded exercise test

Unless your health care provider orders it or you participate in a research study like ours, the graded exercise test is not a test you can or should do. If your exercise provider is affiliated with a rehabilitation setting, she or he can work with your primary care provider or cardiologist to order a graded exercise test because it is the gold standard test for assessing aerobic fitness. Otherwise, your exercise provider should resort to the tests below. Our research studies have shown that the graded exercise test is feasible and safe for people with Alzheimer's dementia. Over the years, we have successfully performed about 500 cycle-based graded exercise tests with older adults who had mild-to-moderate Alzheimer's dementia.

Shuttle walk test

Your exercise provider who is trained to do the shuttle walk test can conduct the test with you because it is an exercise test for the field. The equipment needed includes a pair of cones (or similar markers), a 33-foot level course (hallway), a heart rate monitor, and a way to play an audio recording of beeps (e.g., an audio player, a smartphone, or a tablet).

The cones are placed 30 feet apart, so you can walk around the cones. At the beginning of the test, you will stand by one cone and walk to the other cone at a speed dictated by the beeps from the audio recording. The goal is to reach the other cone before a beep is heard. The test begins with a countdown of beeps; at this point, you walk to and around the other cone to wait for the next beep before returning to the starting cone. When three beeps occur, the pace quickens, so you must walk faster. Your exercise provider can give you verbal reminders coinciding with the beeps such as 1) "Stop" when you arrive at a cone before the beep; 2) "Go" when the single beep for walking sounds; and, 3) "Walk faster now" when the triple beeps sound.

The shuttle walk test has 12 stages, with a minimum walking speed of 1.2 miles per hour and a maximum speed of 5.3 miles per hour. Laps are tallied during the test, and total walking distance is recorded. As with the graded exercise test, the resting and peak heart rates recorded during the shuttle walk test are used to individualize exercise intensity. The limitation of the shuttle walk test is that your heart rhythm will not be recorded as the graded exercise test, so it cannot uncover any unknown heart conditions.

Six-minute walk test

Your exercise provider can also conduct the six-minute walk test with you if the shuttle walk test is too hard to do for some reasons. The equipment needed includes a heart rate monitor, a timer, and a length of hard, flat surface such as a hallway. You will walk on the hard, flat surface for as far as possible for six minutes. The test is self-paced and allows you to take a rest. Because it is self-paced, peak heart rates may not reach the level seen in the graded exercise test and the shuttle walk test. In our studies, we marked a 75-foot long hallway and have our participants walk back and forth from one end to another for six minutes, so we can easily measure how far they have walked in six minutes.

What Is the Target Exercise Dose?

Now that you have completed our Approach AD S.A.F.E.ly™ pre-exercise health screening, you are ready to design your aerobic exercise program. Let us first look at your target aerobic exercise dose.

We recommend that you participate in 150 minutes of moderate-intensity aerobic exercise a week as the target exercise dose for promoting brain health, preventing AD, and treating AD symptoms. We further recommend three times a week for exercise frequency and no more than 60 minutes per exercise session. Our recommendations are based on our own research findings and the current scientific evidence.

Table 7.1. Examples for Achieving the Recommended Dose

Moderate intensity	Times per Week	Minutes per Session
Low frequency / High duration	3	50
Moderate frequency / Moderate duration	4	37
High frequency / How duration	5	30

Systematic reviews and meta-analyses have shown that you need to exercise about one hour three times a week or six months to prevent Alzheimer's dementia. To treat cognitive decline in Alzheimer's dementia, you need, on average, 45 minutes of moderate-intensity aerobic exercise for an average of 137 minutes per week. The World Health Organization recommends moderate-intensity aerobic exercise for at least 150 minutes per week, vigorous-intensity aerobic exercise for 75 minutes a week, or a combination of the two, plus muscle-strengthening training two or more times a week for brain health.

Our recommendation can be considered as the minimum amount of aerobic exercise you need. Once you have increased your aerobic fitness over time, you can consider increasing your exercise dose slowly and as tolerated by increasing the frequency to four to seven days a week. While more exercise is better for overall health and other conditions, it remains unknown if this is also true for AD prevention and treatment. The current evidence suggests not to exceed 60 minutes of exercise in a given exercise session for optimal health benefits.

How Do I Use the FITT-VP Principle?

Now that you have a clear idea of the target aerobic exercise dose, it does not mean that you should start at this dose of exercise right away. In our studies, it usually takes seven to eight weeks for our participants to reach this target level, a rate that has helped them adjust to exercise and enjoy it.

The FITT-VP Principle

At this point, if you begin to have questions like "What should I do to eventually reach the target aerobic exercise dose?" "What is my moderate intensity?" or "What mode of exercise is best for me?" you are on the right track. You can follow a commonly used strategy from the ACSM known as the FITT-VP principle. The FITT-VP acronym represents Frequency (how often), Intensity (how hard), Time (duration, or how long), Type (mode or what kind), Volume (how much or amount—a combination of Frequency, Intensity, and Time), and Progression (advancement).

The FITT-VP principle ensures that you are not overworking and are gradually progressing or increasing exercise to the target level. The FITT-VP principle is another way to further ensure that you reach your target exercise dose safely and that you are in the best possible position to achieve your exercise goals. Following the FITT-VP principle, our research participants have rarely had a problem during or after aerobic exercise.

Moderate Intensity

A common concern among people who just start to exercise is not knowing how hard to exercise. The good news is that there are several ways to define exercise intensity, including objective methods such as heart rate reserve and age-predicted max heart rate to calculate your target heart rate or subjective indicators such as the rating of perceived exertion scale, talk test, and signs and symptoms of overexertion.

Objective moderate intensity

If your exercise provider has assessed your resting and peak heart rate using one of the three aerobic fitness tests described previously, you can determine your heart rate reserve yourself. Heart rate reserve is the difference between your peak and resting heart rates. Because 40% to 60% of heart rate reserve is considered moderate intensity, you can then calculate the heart rates for this range and add them to your resting heart rate to get your target heart rate zone for moderate intensity.

Let us take Kayla's example. Kayla took the six-minute walk test with her exercise provider. Her resting and peak heart rates were 70 and 100 beats per minute, respectively, so her heart rate reserve is 30 (= 100 - 70). Forty percent of her heart rate reserve is 12 (= 30 x 40%), and 60% of her heart rate reserve is 18 (= 30 x 60%). Adding these to her resting heart rate of 70 gives her a target heart rate zone of 82 to 88 beats per minute for her moderate intensity. Another example is for calculating your target hear rate zone is provided in Figure 7.1.

However, keep in mind that the six-minute walk test is a submaximal test instead of a true peak test like the graded exercise test or shuttle walk test. This means that her peak heart rate obtained from the six-minute walk test is likely lower than her true peak heart rate derived from the graded exercise test or shuttle walk test. Is this ok then? Yes, it is because a low estimate means that the exercise will be less challenging for Kayla, which is perfectly fine if Kayla just started to exercise. With aerobic exercise, Kayla's heart and lungs will be conditioned. Hence, regular aerobic fitness assessment such as every six months is needed to recalculate her moderate intensity.

The Alzheimer's Rx: Aerobic Exercise

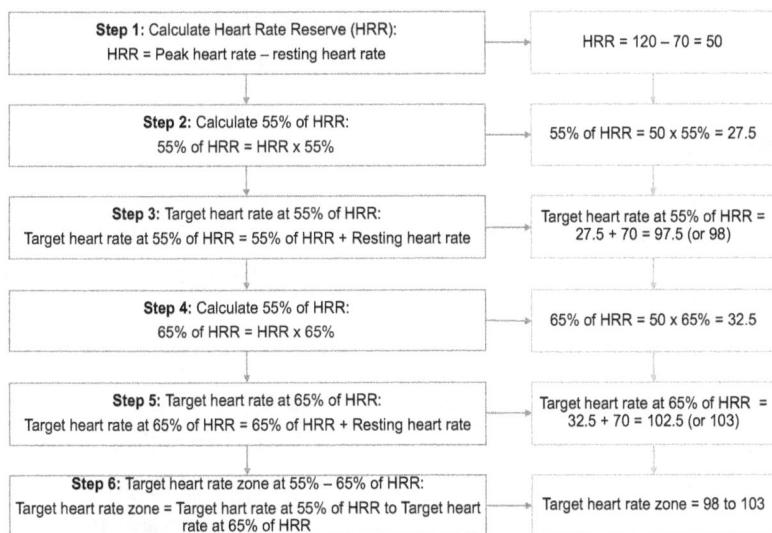

Step 1: Calculate Heart Rate Reserve (HRR): HRR = Peak heart rate – resting heart rate	HRR = 120 – 70 = 50
Step 2: Calculate 55% of HRR: 55% of HRR = HRR x 55%	55% of HRR = 50 x 55% = 27.5
Step 3: Target heart rate at 55% of HRR: Target heart rate at 55% of HRR = 55% of HRR + Resting heart rate	Target heart rate at 55% of HRR = 27.5 + 70 = 97.5 (or 98)
Step 4: Calculate 55% of HRR: 65% of HRR = HRR x 65%	65% of HRR = 50 x 65% = 32.5
Step 5: Target heart rate at 65% of HRR: Target heart rate at 65% of HRR = 65% of HRR + Resting heart rate	Target heart rate at 65% of HRR = 32.5 + 70 = 102.5 (or 103)
Step 6: Target heart rate zone at 55% – 65% of HRR: Target heart rate zone = Target hart rate at 55% of HRR to Target heart rate at 65% of HRR	Target heart rate zone = 98 to 103

Figure 7.1. **Example of Calculating the Target Heart Rate Zone from Heart Rate Reserve** (based on peak heart rate of 120 beats per minute from an aerobic fitness test & resting heart rate of 70 beats per minute)

You can also use the age-predicted max heart rate method. It requires you to predict your maximum heart rate using the following formula: maximal heart rate = 220 – age in years or = 208 – (0.7 x age in years). You will then calculate moderate intensity as 50% to 70% of your maximum heart rate. As you see, the age-based formula is not an individualized method because people of the same age will have the same maximum heart estimate when in fact they could differ considerably in their aerobic fitness. This method should only be used when the heart rate reserve method is not feasible and is used jointly with the subjective methods of moderate intensity discussed later. You should not use the age-predicted max heart rate method if you take medications that slow your heart rate, such as beta-blockers.

Subjective moderate intensity

Aerobic fitness testing may simply not be possible for some people. In this case, you will rely on your subjective perception to gauge exercise intensity. You can use three tools: The rating of perceived exertion scale (how hard you feel you are exercising); the talk test (ability to speak a sentence during exercise); and signs and symptoms of overexertion (e.g., amount of sweating, and breathing difficulty).

You can choose from several commercially available rating of perceived exertion scale scales. The most commonly used is the Borg 6–20 scale. Some landmarks on the Borg 6–20 scale include: 6 = no exertion; 11 = fairly light; 13 = somewhat hard; 15 = hard; and 20 = maximum. We consider 12 and 13 moderate intensity in our research studies. Another scale is the 10-point scale, which defines moderate intensity as three or four. The rating of perceived exertion scale also has narrative descriptors and facial expressions that go along with each number, so you can use the number, narrative descriptions, and/or facial expressions to rate your exercise exertion.

When you exercise, moderate intensity can also be described as a "conversational pace" on the talk test, in which you would be able to talk or hold a conversation without becoming breathless. If you find yourself pausing your conversation in order to catch breath, you are working harder than moderate intensity. On the other hand, if you can still sing, then you are exercising at a lower than moderate intensity.

Signs and symptoms can also help gauge your exercise intensity. During moderate-intensity exercise, you will sweat and breathe harder. However, if you are sweating profusely and have symptoms such as lightheadedness, dizziness, nausea, or heart palpitations, you may be exercising too hard. If you do not work up a sweat or breathe harder, then you probably are exercising below moderate intensity.

Your FITT-VP

Consider starting with 45 to 60 minutes of low-intensity aerobic exercise (40% of heart rate reserve or rating of perceived exertion 8) weekly, that is, 15 to 20 minutes per session, three times per week in the first week. You can gradually build up to 150 minutes of moderate-intensity aerobic exercise per week over several weeks. The adjustment period depends on how your body responds to aerobic exercise, but consider giving it five to eight weeks, especially if you have not been exercising regularly. This adjustment reflects the general principle "start low and increase slowly over time" described in Chapter 4.

The three-times-a-week frequency can be set up on alternate days such as Monday-Wednesday-Friday or Tuesday-Thursday-Saturday, which will allow you to recuperate between exercise sessions while setting up an exercise structure you can continue to build on. An exercise program that is more frequent may be too burdensome when you are just starting out, while less frequency could be demotivating and feel like you are not doing much.

If you can complete the first week (three sessions) as planned, in the second week, you can either increase the session's duration by five minutes or increase the intensity by boosting your exercise heart rate by 5% of heart rate reserve or one rating of perceived exertion. However, do not increase both session duration and intensity at the same time. If your second week or sessions 4–6 went as planned, you can again increase your session duration by five minutes or the intensity by 5% heart rate or one rating of perceived exertion increase in the third week or session 7–9. Continue to do this until you reach the target 150-minute moderate-intensity weekly dose (Table 7.2).

Another way to adjust your exercise dose is to increase the intensity by boosting your exercise heart rate by 5% or one rating of perceived exertion per week while keeping the session duration the same until you reach the target moderate intensity. Then you can prolong your session duration by five minutes per week until you reach 50 minutes of moderate-intensity aerobic exercise a session. Similarly, you can keep your intensity the same while increasing your session durations weekly until you reach 50 minutes per session. Then you can increase the exercise intensity weekly until you achieve moderate intensity.

Table 7.2. Example of Exercise Progression and Dose

Week number	Session number	Moderate Intensity		Duration at moderate intensity
		Target heart rate zone at % heart rate reserve	Borg 6-20 rating of perceived exertion scale	
1	1 – 3	Target heart rate zone at 40% – 50%	11 – 12	30
2	4 – 6	Target heart rate zone at 40% – 50%	11 – 12	35
3	7 – 9	Target heart rate zone at 45% – 55%	11 – 12	35
4	10 – 12	Target heart rate zone at 45% – 55%	11 – 12	40
5	13 – 15	Target heart rate zone at 50% – 60%	12 – 13	40
6	16 – 18	Target heart rate zone at 50% – 60%	12 – 13	45
7	19 – 21	Target heart rate zone at 55% – 65%	13 – 14	45
8+	22+	Target heart rate zone at 55% – 65%	13 – 14	50

Note. See Figure 7.1 to learn how to calculate target heart rate zone at different heart rate reserve.

Exercise Mode Selection

Now that you have seen several different ways to go about reaching the target exercise dose, you can build your own exercise that will work the best for you. The next step is to determine what kind of aerobic exercise is the best for you. In Chapter 4, we listed a variety of aerobic exercises from which to choose based on your preferences and circumstances. Cycling is our preferred mode for older adults with Alzheimer's dementia because it is safe and not weight-bearing, and does not require previous knowledge and experience. If you do not have access to a cycle or gym, walking is a good choice.

Time to Exercise

Finding the time to exercise is a common challenge for those who are thinking of starting an exercise program. You may have seen many young and working people choose to exercise in the early morning before work or heard that exercise in the morning is a great way to jumpstart your metabolism. However, the truth is that there is no reliable evidence to suggest that you will exercise more effectively at certain times of a day. However, the time of the day can influence how you feel or respond when exercising. Truthfully, the most important thing is to choose a time of the day that works the best for you and try to be consistent with it so exercise becomes part of your daily routine.

Based on our experiences and the current understanding of circadian rhythms, we recommend that older adults with Alzheimer's dementia do aerobic exercise in the late morning or mid-afternoon, if possible. This is because the circadian clock anticipates and adapts the body to the different phases of the day, such as regulating sleep patterns, eating behavior, alertness, hormone release, blood pressure, and body temperature. In particular, humans are thought to be the most alert in the mid-to-late morning and have the best coordination and fastest reaction times in the early afternoon. While stress hormones such as cortisol are at their highest and blood pressures increase most rapidly in the early morning, blood pressures are highest in the evening. Because high blood pressure is common in people with Alzheimer's dementia, it may be best to avoid exercise in early morning and evening.

Another reason for our late morning and early-to-mid afternoon recommendation is to reduce the chance that behavioral and psychological symptoms of dementia will manifest during exercise. As detailed in Chapter 9, these symptoms tend to occur in the late evening, which could make exercise engagement less effective. On the other hand, exercise has been shown to reduce these symptoms.

Returning to Exercise After Absence

Despite your best intention, it is very likely that your exercise routine gets interrupted for weeks. Some common interruptions among our research participants have been extended vacations, acute illness, a flare-up of a chronic condition, or medical clearance needed for evaluating a new sign or symptom. If you have not been exercising for two weeks or more, then you should return to your aerobic exercise at a lower dose. One way to re-start exercise is to revert back to the exercise dose you were doing by the number of weeks you were absent before you stopped exercising. For example, if you were in your 12th week of exercise and missed two weeks, you can re-start at the exercise dose of week 10 (= 12 weeks – 2 weeks); if you missed three weeks, then re-start at the dose for week 9 (= 12 weeks – 3 weeks); and so on.

Key Messages

- Use our S.A.F.E. Tool to conduct pre-exercise health screening before starting an aerobic exercise program.
- Exercise readiness can be assessed using the Physical Activity Readiness Questionnaire, the 2015 ACSM Preparticipation

Health Screening Algorithm, or the Exercise Assessment and Screening for You.

- Medical evaluation is needed if indicated by the exercise readiness tool or if you have questions about your ability to exercise safely.
- Aerobic fitness can be evaluated using a graded exercise test, the shuttle walk test, or the 6-minute walk test.
- The target dose for preventing and treating AD is 150 minutes of moderate-intensity aerobic exercise per week. However, you need to progress to this dose over five to eight weeks to ensure exercise safety. A good starting dose is 45 to 60 minutes of low-intensity aerobic exercise weekly, three times a week, for 15 to 20 minutes per session.
- Moderate intensity can be personalized based on your heart rate reserve obtained from an aerobic fitness test. If you cannot take part in an aerobic fitness test, you can use the subjective method or couple the subjective method with an age-based formula to determine your own moderate intensity.
- The Approach AD S.A.F.E.ly™ protocol uses the FITT-VP principle to personalize your exercise program and select your preferred exercise type. The best time for exercise is late morning and early-to-mid afternoon for older adults with Alzheimer's dementia.

The Beginning Scenarios

Now let us return to the four scenarios at the beginning of this chapter. Marie's concern about exercise safety is often reported as the No. 1 barrier to exercise. The 2015 ACSM Preparticipation Health Screening Algorithm or Exercise Assessment and Screening for You tool can put her mind at ease.

In John's case, we discovered an unknown heart condition during exercise testing, although he was initially medically cleared by his primary care provider. The good news is that John's blood pressure, heart rate, and heart rhythm were all normal, and he had no symptoms. While such an occurrence is rare, it has happened a few times in our 15 years of exercise research. A colleague had remarked that this is the case in which participating in a research study may actually save a life. John then underwent another exercise test in his cardiologist's office and had a stent placed. His cardiologist cleared him to continue with our study.

Another common challenge in pre-exercise health screening pertains to potential chest pain, as in Frank's case. Given the impact of AD on communication, it is important to have a complete medical history, be able to ask questions in several different ways, and use a variety of descriptive terms to evaluate symptoms. The Exercise Assessment and Screening for You tool could be the most useful in this case. Even when aerobic exercise is considered safe initially, there may be times when exercise is not appropriate, so ongoing monitoring of exercise safety is critical, which will be fully described in the next chapter.

In James' case, Jesse followed our Approach AD S.A.F.E.ly™ pre-exercise health screening, which helped him identify chest tightness. James had been attributing this symptom to heartburn or lack of rest. He did not realize that it could indicate cardiovascular conditions. His case further illustrates the importance of timely communication between you and your exercise provider to ensure and timely disease treatment and safe exercise participation.

Chapter 8

How Do I Ensure Safety During Aerobic Exercise?

" *I am starting my third week in aerobic exercise at my health club. I just get on the bike and immediately go to 60 revolutions per minute at a resistance of five for 30 minutes; as soon as the 30 minutes are up, I hop off the bike to meet up with my friends to play cards. I do not have any complaints. I work up a great sweat and feel like I am accomplishing a lot, but I sure do get dizzy when I get off the bike. I wish I could change that."*
~Fred, an exerciser

"*I have been supervising James' exercise program for the past four months. James is 77 and has Alzheimer's dementia. At the beginning of the program, I noticed that the target heart rate zones I calculated for moderate-intensity matched really well with his rating of perceived exertion. However, in the last month, he reports perceived exertion of 14 to 15, even though his heart rate did not change. Is this normal?"* ~Donald, an exercise provider

---

"I am just starting the first week of my exercise program. I read how to calculate my heart rate zones to find my target intensity. The one that looked the easiest for me was based on my age. It said that, in order to reach moderate intensity, I need to work out at a heart rate of 90 to 105. However, when I exercise, it is very hard for me to even reach a heart rate of 90. Did I do something wrong?" ~Jane, an exerciser

---

"I have been exercising regularly now for four months. In fact, I have not missed one session since I started, and I feel great! I have more energy than ever, and my doctor says my blood pressure is the best he has seen in years! Recently, I caught a pretty bad cold. It was hard for me to get going this morning, but I do not want to miss my exercise session today. Is it appropriate for me to exercise when I have a cold? In fact, I guess I am not totally sure when it is appropriate to avoid exercise." ~Fran, an exerciser

You have read commonly asked questions that come up once an exercise program has begun. You may relate to some of these testimonials or may have some of your own. Now that you have determined that it is safe for you to exercise, performed a test of aerobic fitness, and created your target heart rate zones for each session, you will learn the "how-to" strategies about engaging in aerobic exercise safely.

In this chapter, you will find out how to use our Approach AD S.A.F.E.ly™ protocol to set up exercise session flow by incorporating a proper warm-up and cool-down. Next, you will become skilled at using our Approach AD S.A.F.E.ly™ exercise response monitoring so you can stay in your target heart rate zone to ensure exercise safety. Last, you will learn how common conditions and their medications can influence your ability to exercise aerobically, and when you should delay, defer, or cancel an exercise session. This chapter addresses you as the person who exercises on your own or as a client of an exercise provider.

How Do I Set up an Exercise Session?

Our Approach AD S.A.F.E.ly™ exercise session flow includes three phases for an exercise session: warm-up, stimulus, and cool-down. Each phase will allow your body to gradually adjust to the stress of exercise.

Warm-Up

Warm-up refers to starting exercise at a low intensity and then gradually increasing the intensity until you reach your target exercise dose. Warm-up prepares your body for the stimulus portion of the exercise session. Specifically, the goal of the warm-up is to allow your body to adapt to the exercise session, improve your exercise performance, and reduce your risk for injury.

Warm-up is very important for both your skeletal and heart muscles. At rest, you have very little blood flow to your skeletal muscles. When you start your warm-up, these blood vessels dilate to increase blood flow to the contracting muscles. The greater the blood flow to your muscles, the better they will perform. Good blood flow also makes it less likely for you to have lactic acid buildup in your muscles, which can result in the "muscle-burning" sensation that often occurs during or after prolonged, high-intensity exercise. In addition, warm-up helps ensure that your heart has an adequate blood supply. If you do vigorous-intensity exercise without warming up, your heart may not have enough blood flow to meet the heart's demand for oxygen.

A proper warm-up includes any type of aerobic exercise that targets the muscles that you will use in the stimulus portion of the aerobic exercise session. Warm-up should start at a low intensity of 20% to 30% heart rate reserve or nine to 11 on the Borg 6–20 Rating of Perceived Exertion (RPE) scale and progress to moderate intensity within five to 10 minutes. For instance, if your intensity goal was 50% to 60% heart rate reserve (or RPE 12 to 13), you may choose to start at 20% heart rate reserve (or RPE 9) and progress by 10% (one RPE) until you reach your target intensity. Now how does this relate to exercising aerobically on the cycle ergometer? Say that you know that, in order to achieve your target heart rate reserve of 50% to 60% (or RPE 13), you use a setting of 60 RPM and resistance of five. For your warm-up, you may choose to start cycling at 30 to 40 revolutions per minute at no resistance. After one minute, increase your speed to 50 revolutions per minute; after two minutes, increase your speed to 60 revolutions per minute to get you to your target speed for the stimulus phase. After three minutes, increase your resistance to two. After four minutes, increase your resistance to four, and at five minutes, move to a resistance of five. Now you would have completed your warm-up within five to 10 minutes and would likely be at the target intensity for the stimulus phase.

Stimulus

The stimulus phase is where the target dose of the aerobic exercise session is performed after warm-up. The goal of the stimulus phase is to maximize the time exercised at your target intensity.

During the stimulus phase, you may need to adjust the settings on your exercise machine or walking speed periodically based on your heart rate or how you feel during the exercise session. If you feel like you are working above your target intensity zone, you should slow your pace or reduce your resistance on your exercise machine in order to stay within your target zone. If you use heart rates to monitor your intensity, there may be times when your heart rate is not quite in your target heart rate zone but you feel like you are exercising at your target level. In this case, listen to your body and stay at the same level. Do not push yourself to get into your target heart rate zone.

Likewise, there may be times when your heart rate may drift above your target heart rate zone. This is most common when you are participating in prolonged aerobic exercise and sweating. In this case, if you feel like you are still exercising at your target RPE, maintain your intensity. However, if you also have a drift in RPE that places you above your target zone, reduce the settings on your machine or slow your walking pace to stay within your target intensity.

Cool-Down

Immediately after the stimulus phase, do a cool-down. The cool-down after the stimulus phase is just as important as warm-up. Remember that immediately after aerobic exercise, your heart is still beating faster, your body temperature is likely higher, and your blood vessels are more dilated than normal. Cool-down allows your body to return to its resting state. Most noticeably with cool-down, your heart rate and blood pressure will return to their resting levels. This gradual return is important to prevent a sudden drop in blood pressure that could lead to dizziness and fainting. Cool-down also helps reduce body heat and any blood lactate that may have formed during the stimulus phase. Lastly, cool-down, like warm-up, helps prevent acute heart problems. Failure to cool down, particularly after moderate- or vigorous-intensity aerobic exercise, increases your risk of fainting, low blood pressure, and heart stress.

Similar to warm-up, cool-down involves performing an aerobic exercise such as walking or cycling at a slow pace for five to 10 minutes. An easy way to cool down would be to reverse what you did during warm-up. For instance, if during the stimulus phase, you were cycling at 60 revolutions per minute and a resistance of five to achieve a heart rate reserve of 50% to 60% (or RPE 13), you would decrease your cycling speed and resistance to reach a lower heart rate reserve of 10% or RPE one per minute, respectively. This could equate to reducing the resistance to four during the first minute, two during the second minute, and zero during the third minute of cool-down. Then you would drop your cycling speed by 10 revolutions per minute until you reach 20 to 30 revolutions per minute, completing the five- to 10-minute phase.

How Should I Monitor Exercise Responses?

Our Approach AD S.A.F.E.ly™ exercise response monitoring uses combined objective and subjective indicators of exercise intensity to evaluate how your body is responding to aerobic exercise during an exercise session. Depending on your specific situation, you may rely on the objective or subjective indicators more than the other. Objective indicators include heart rate, and signs such as breathing, sweating pattern and amount, and skin color and temperature. Subjective indicators are your perceived exertion, ability to talk a sentence, and symptoms such as dizziness and discomfort.

Heart Rate

There are three general ways to easily monitor your heart rate during exercise: 1) Some exercise machines have sensors on the handles that measure your heart rate if you grasp them for a brief time, 2) Manually check your heart rate, or 3) Use a commercially available heart rate monitor. There are pros and cons to each.

Several exercise machines, including most recumbent stationary cycles, have built-in handgrip monitors to detect heart rate during exercise, which allows you to check your heart rate in real-time. You do not have to buy or wear additional equipment. However, the accuracy of the handgrip monitors depends on the contact between your hand and the device, and the sensitivity of the monitors can lessen over time. In general, treadmills might have the most inaccurate handgrip sensors, while stationary cycles and elliptical machines may be more accurate.

Commercially available heart rate monitors are generally either chest-strapped or wrist-based. For the chest-strap heart rate monitors, a wireless sensor on a chest strap detects your heart rate electronically and sends the data to a wristwatch-style receiver for display. Chest-strap monitors provide the most accurate heart-rate results but require you to get used to the routine of putting on the chest strap. Wrist-based heart rate monitors have an optical sensor built into the back of the wrist unit's watchband or case that detects your pulse. Although heart rate monitor watches are slightly less accurate, wrist-based models avoid the potential discomfort and additional pre-workout time associated with putting on the chest strap.

If you do not want to use heart rate monitors but still want to periodically assess your heart rate, you can do so manually. One method you can use is to measure your pulse manually on the inside of your wrist for 15 seconds. Once you get this 15-second heart rate, multiply it by four to get your heart rate in beats per minute. Manual heart rates can be problematic for treadmill-based exercise but are less so with cycling.

During exercise, if you monitor your heart rate, it should increase as exercise intensity increases and plateau once you reach your steady-state or target intensity level. Your heart rate should remain relatively constant as long as you do not increase your pace or adjust exercise intensity. However, remember that your heart rate can slowly drift above your target heart rate zone during prolonged aerobic exercise.

Perceived Exertion

Several RPE scales are commercially available. The most commonly used are the Borg 6-20 scale and the 10-point modified scale. In our research studies, we asked participants to rate their exertion every five minutes. You may also want to use this strategy in your exercise program. However, you may also choose to do this just once in the middle of your session. There is no one perfect strategy or timing to assess your perceived exertion. We advise adopting a routine that works best for you. The most important thing is to be aware of how your body is feeling while you exercise so you can respond accordingly.

Accurate depiction of the RPE is important, particularly if you plan to use RPE as a primary indicator of exercise intensity. However, it is not uncommon that people will over- or under-estimate their RPE. While over-estimation is less of a concern, underestimation, when exercise intensity is actually higher, may increase your risk for adverse events and injuries.

In our research studies, we have found that about a third of the participants could not understand RPE or use it accurately (use it to rate pain or pick out a random rating). Hence, we assessed participants' ability to use RPE accurately by comparing the ratings to heart rate and talk test, got to know how they use RPE, and always combined RPE with the other indicators of exercise intensity.

Talk Test

The talk test is another subjective way to gauge your exercise intensity. If you are exercising with a friend, try to talk and monitor your speech patterns. For instance, you may choose to tell them about something you recently did, heard, or read about. If you are able to talk easily without pausing to catch your breath or can sing a song, you are working below moderate intensity. However, if you are pausing several times during your sentence to catch your breath, you are working harder than moderate intensity. One or two breaths per sentence are about right if you are working at moderate intensity. If you are exercising by yourself, you may choose to recite a passage, read a sentence, or sing a song to yourself to gauge your exercise intensity.

In our research, we have found that some participants did not like to talk during exercise. In this event, we have written a four-sentence script on the back of our RPE scale and asked our participants to read it to us when we did the talk test. As with using RPE, there is no perfect time to use the talk test, but you should make it a habit to check your breathing every time you talk during exercise. Over time, it will become part of your exercise routine.

Exertion Signs and Symptoms

It is important to pay close attention to the changes in your breathing, skin color, and sweating during aerobic exercise to see if you are responding normally to exercise. A normal response to aerobic exercise is an increase in your breathing rate and depth as your exercise intensity increases. This respiratory response, particularly your breathing rate, may be greater if you have other conditions such as asthma or chronic obstructive pulmonary disease. In these cases, you may have shortness of breath during exercise, so make sure you bring your inhaler to your exercise sessions to prevent a full-blown attack.

Moderate-intensity exercise causes a change in blood distribution. For example, the blood flow to your skeletal muscles and skin increases. The increase in skin blood flow leads to sweating and redness (which is a good thing).

While we have used all these methods to monitor exercise responses in our studies, you can pick one as your primary method. The pros and cons of each method is summarized in Table 8.1.

Table 8.1. Comparison of Tools for Monitoring Exercise Response

Tool	Pros	Cons
Heart rate	Objective and accurate Continuous feedback if using a heart rate monitor	Affected by medications
Rating of perceived exertion	Quick and easy Different cues (e.g., numbers, facial expressions)	Misinterpretation of cues Over- or under-rating
Talk test	Quick and easy Relating well to rating of perceived exertion	Challenging to people who are naturally quiet
Signs and symptoms	Effective for assessing physiological response	Being self-aware or in tune with self

How Does Exercise Response Change?

Improvements in aerobic fitness often occur at the same time as enhanced efficiency of your cardiovascular, pulmonary, and metabolic systems. Aerobic exercise increases blood plasma volume, blood flow, and the amount of blood your heart ejects per heartbeat. In addition, your heart may undergo changes with equal increases in chamber volume and muscle mass. The increase in the amount of blood your heart ejects per heartbeat is a sign of greater cardiac efficiency and will make your heart stronger. As a result of these changes to your heart, your resting and peak exercise heart rates can decrease from what they were before you started your aerobic exercise program.

Likewise, when you improve your aerobic fitness, you breathe more efficiently, causing your breathing rate to decrease at rest and during low-intensity exercise. In addition, with increased blood plasma volume, delivery of blood to the skin, and sweat gland enlargement, you may sweat more during exercise. This is why you need more water during exercise, regardless of the weather or feeling of thirst.

These changes may affect your exercise responses. For instance, over time, it may become more challenging to achieve a target heart rate zone than it was when you first started your aerobic exercise program. When this happens, you need to re-establish your target heart rate zone, which is why we recommend regular aerobic fitness testing, e.g., every six months. If you notice that you are having a tough time reaching your target heart rate zones and cannot retest your aerobic fitness and recalculate your target heart rate zones, you can rely on RPE as a primary gauge of your intensity, along with the talk test, signs, and symptoms.

If you use RPE as a primary tool to monitor your exercise intensity, the RPE at a given exercise intensity may also change. For instance, say you started your aerobic exercise program at resistance level two to reach RPE 12. After 12 weeks of regular aerobic exercise, to reach an RPE of 12, you may be cycling at a resistance of six. In addition, when using the talk test, you will notice as the aerobic exercise program progresses, it will be easier to talk without becoming breathless. Therefore, you may need to adjust the settings on the cycle to achieve the target RPE levels.

How Can Diseases Affect Exercise Safety?

Several conditions are very common in older adults, such as high blood pressure, type 2 diabetes, chronic pain, and depression, which we frequently observe in our research participants. These conditions and their medications may affect exercise responses and safety. Please note that not all medications within a given class are discussed here; we are featuring only those that are common and can substantially affect your ability to exercise aerobically and your safety.

High Blood Pressure and its Medications

Over 63% of people aged 65 to 74 years and over 72% of those older than 75 in the United States have high blood pressure and/or are taking blood pressure medications. Regular, moderate-to-vigorous intensity aerobic exercise can reduce blood pressure by, on average, five to seven mmHg within eight to 12 weeks.

If you have high blood pressure, monitor your blood pressure before and after exercise, because blood pressure readings of 200/100 mmHg are a reason to avoid exercise, as discussed in Chapter 7. If you have high blood pressure, take your blood pressure medication before exercising to ensure your blood pressure is in the safe range. Taking your blood pressure after exercise will show whether your blood pressure has returned to normal. In our research studies, we logged pre- and post-exercise blood pressure readings for our participants. Seeing the positive changes in their resting blood pressures have motivated them to continue their aerobic exercise program.

Two common types of high blood pressure medications are beta-blockers and calcium channel blockers. In different ways, both relieve stress on your heart by slowing heart rate and the force with which the heart muscle contracts to lower blood pressure. During exercise, these medications can prevent excessive increases in heart rate, so you may not see a normal heart rate response. This means that heart rate cannot be used accurately for monitoring exercise responses if you only based your exercise intensity on the age-predicted max heart rate method described in Chapter 7. However, if you have performed an aerobic fitness test while on a beta-blocker, your peak heart rate can be accurately determined and used for calculating your target heart zones. Despite this, you also want to use the RPE, talk test, signs, and symptoms as indicators of your exercise intensity, because your target heart rate zones may be too narrow, e.g., having a zone of only a few heartbeats apart, which makes it difficult to stay in zones.

Diabetes and its Medications

In 2015, the Centers for Disease Control and Prevention estimated that 30.3 million Americans, or 9.4% of the U.S. population, have diabetes. The occurrence of diabetes increases with age. Four percent of adults aged 18 to 44 have diabetes, while 17% of those 45 to 64 and 25% of those 65 years and older have it. As with high blood pressure, aerobic exercise is an important treatment for diabetes because it boosts insulin sensitivity. Insulin action in muscle and liver can change with exercise, which increases muscle use of blood sugar up to fivefold. After exercise, blood sugar uptake by muscles remains high for as long as 48 hours if you exercise at least 30 minutes. Improvements in insulin action may last for 24 hours after shorter durations (about 20 minutes) if the intensity is increased intermittently. Even 60 minutes of low-intensity aerobic exercise increases insulin action in people with obesity and diabetes for at least 24 hours.

If you have diabetes, there is a safe blood sugar range before starting an exercise session: ideally 90 to 250 mg/dL (5.0 and 13.9 mmol/L). You may need to eat some carbohydrates before exercise, depending on if and when you take insulin, the timing of your exercise, your starting blood sugar levels, and durations of aerobic exercise (e.g., 30 minutes or longer). Therefore, if you have diabetes (especially type 1), it is important to check blood sugar before and after each exercise session. As a general rule, do not start exercising if your blood sugar is less than 90 mg/dL until you have had 15 to 30 g (e.g., one or two choices) of fast-acting carbohydrates. In addition, it is important to time your exercise sessions so you can ensure safety if one of your diabetes medications is insulin. Avoid aerobic exercise at peak insulin action. Peak insulin action varies depending on the type of insulin used. Lastly, if you have specific questions related to the timing of exercise relative to your insulin routine, discuss with your primary care provider or diabetes educator.

Pain and Painkillers

Advanced age increases the risk of certain health conditions that can cause chronic pain, such as arthritis, osteoporosis, peripheral vascular disorders, and nerve pain. In the past, people with chronic pain were told to rest. However, the general advice now is to keep active, whether to relieve pain directly or to combat problems linked to it. Aerobic exercise can be an important part of the treatment plan for chronic pain because of its painkilling effects and improved physical fitness, which reduces stress on joints and promotes anti-inflammatory effects and endorphin release.

Some pain medications can affect your ability to exercise. Pain medications are often classified into three categories: nonsteroidal anti-inflammatory drugs (e.g., ibuprofen), acetaminophen, and opioids. Both nonsteroidal anti-inflammatory drugs and acetaminophen can make aerobic exercise easier by reducing inflammation or blocking pain without affecting your ability to exercise.

Opioids such as codeine, morphine, oxycodone, and hydrocodone have been shown to decrease exercise performance by delaying reaction time, causing sedation, and reducing cardiorespiratory drive. Specifically, opioids slow your heart rate and respiratory rate. As a result, they can reduce your peak oxygen consumption, limiting your ability to exercise aerobically. Opioids can also make you fatigue quicker than usual, particularly during aerobic exercise; as a result, you may think you are exercising harder than normal. Also, you need to consider the type of exercise you do if you take opioids because people who take opioids fall more often than those taking other types of pain medications. Therefore, stationary types of aerobic exercise (e.g., recumbent cycling) are often a safer choice if you take opioids, particularly if you have noticeable balance problems or a history of falls.

Depression and Antidepressants

Currently, one in 10 Americans have depression. Research over the past two decades has shown that aerobic exercise helps improve depression and prevent it from coming back. However, if you have depression, you may find it difficult to start and sustain an exercise routine. Your motivation to exercise may be affected by depressive symptoms such as fatigue, trouble making decisions, low self-esteem, loss of interest and pleasure, and poor sleep. In particular, people with depression, anxiety, and low fitness may find it difficult to exercise. Because of exercise's antidepressant effects, strategies to sustain exercise are needed for people who do not.

Some antidepressants, such as selective serotonin reuptake inhibitors (SSRIs), can cause a "drowsy" effect, which can reduce your ability to exercise. However, current research investigating the effects of SSRIs on fatigue during aerobic exercise have produced mixed results, with some studies showing that SSRIs have a negative influence and others showing no effect. If you take an SSRI that makes you drowsy, you may think you are exercising harder than you really are—especially if you exercise for longer than 30 minutes.

When Do I Change a Session?

Regardless of whether you are just starting exercise or exercise regularly, your health can change from one day to another. As you begin to notice the benefits of regular exercise, you may be increasingly motivated to continue exercising, even during uncertain or bad times. However, there are times when it is best to delay, defer, or even cancel an exercise session.

Reasons to Delay

High blood pressure

If you have high blood pressure, measure your blood pressure before and after exercise. If your systolic blood pressure is 200 mmHg or higher and/or your diastolic blood pressure is 100 mmHg or higher, do not start exercising. Sit calmly and quietly for five minutes and then recheck. If your blood pressure drops below these thresholds, begin your warm-up; however, if it stays at or above this threshold, do not exercise that day.

Abnormal blood sugar level

If you have diabetes and your blood sugar level is less than 90 mg/dL, wait to start your warm-up until you have had 15 to 30 g (e.g., one or two choices) of fast-acting carbohydrates. Then wait 10 minutes and recheck your blood sugar. Once it is above 90 mg/dL, begin your warm-up. However, if your blood sugar level is 250 mg/dL or higher, avoid exercising until it drops below this threshold. The time it may take for your blood sugar to fall under this threshold may vary based on the timing of last carbohydrate intake and medication use.

Reasons to Defer

If you have one of several common health conditions, you should not exercise. These conditions include active infection, chest pain, and muscle soreness or pain. Also, there may be times where your exercise environment (e.g., temperature, humidity) is not safe to exercise.

Infection

Common contagious infections, especially during winter, are the common cold and influenza. If you have an active infection or feel ill, do not exercise that day.

Chest pain

In Chapter 7, you learned about some signs and symptoms of chest pain. During the Approach AD S.A.F.E.ly™ pre-exercise health screening, you may not have signs or symptoms of heart disease; however, you may not have had a high enough workload during activities of daily living to recognize signs and symptoms of chest pain. These signs and symptoms can develop before, during, or after exercise. If you experience chest pain, avoid exercise and strenuous physical activity until your primary care provider or cardiologist has seen and cleared you to resume exercise.

Muscle soreness or pain

Some problems that can occur during exercise are delayed muscle soreness or a flare-up of an orthopedic condition such as arthritis. Do not exercise on days when you have a flare-up. Wait until you feel better to resume your exercise program.

Environment

Your environment can also affect your ability to exercise. Avoid exercising outdoors on days when the weather makes roads slippery, which increases your risk for falls. Also, avoid exercising outdoors in extreme cold, heat, or humidity. If you do exercise on these days, ensure that you do it inside a safe, temperature-controlled environment.

There may be times when you develop signs and symptoms of cardiovascular or metabolic diseases. In these cases, it is important to stop exercising and call 911 or your primary care provider immediately.

Reasons to Cancel

Your health is constantly changing, and unfortunately, some changes may require you to postpone your exercise program. Three of the most common reasons to postpone are the worsening of a heart condition that does not get better with medications, a new disease that can be aggravated by exercise, or new signs and symptoms that have not been evaluated by your health care provider. Likewise, major surgeries require re-clearance by your health care provider to re-start your exercise program. You should also postpone if you have behavioral and psychological symptoms or worsening psychiatric conditions that cannot be controlled.

Key Messages

- Our Approach AD S.A.F.E.ly™ exercise session setup includes a warm-up (five to 10 minutes at low intensity), stimulus (target exercise intensity and duration), and cool-down (five to 10 minutes at low intensity) phase.
- Our Approach AD S.A.F.E.ly™ exercise response monitoring uses combined objective such as heart rate and subjective indicators such as RPE, talk test, signs, and symptoms.
- High blood pressure, diabetes, chronic pain, and depression are common and can affect your exercise ability and responses. Aerobic exercise is an established treatment for these conditions
- If you take high blood pressure medications that affect heart rate, such as a beta-blocker, use your heart rate from the aerobic fitness test and subjective methods for determining exercise intensity.
- Insulin for diabetes or opioids for chronic pain may affect your ability to exercise safely. The timing of your exercise may vary, depending on the type of insulin you take.

- Health is fluid and can change by the day. It is important to know when to delay, defer, or cancel an exercise session to ensure safety.

The Beginning Scenarios

Now, let us return to the four scenarios at the beginning of this chapter. Fred forgot about two components of his workout: the warm-up and cool down. Because Fred immediately stops exercising once his 30-minute workout is over, he may be experiencing a drop in blood pressure, particularly when he stands up from his cycle. This could cause his dizziness. If Fred ends his workout with a cool-down, his blood pressure will gradually return to his resting level, which can prevent dizziness.

One of the great things about aerobic exercise is the positive way it changes the heart. The heart becomes more efficient and does not have to beat as many times. However, this can affect your heart rate zones, as we saw in the case of Donald's client. Because his heart is becoming more efficient, Donald's client has to work harder than he did initially to reach his target heart rate zone. As a result, there is a difference between the target heart rate zone and perceived exertion. This is one reason to retest your aerobic fitness periodically.

In the case of Jane, a couple of reasons were behind her inability to reach her target heart rate zone. First, she miscalculated her target heart rate zone. Second, she was on a medication that is blunting her heart rate response to exercise. However, if she had calculated her target heart rate zones accurately and was not on a medication that affects her heart rate, she should ask her primary care provider why her heart rate is not increasing when she is exercising, despite her feeling of working hard.

In our last case, it was great to see that Fran has not missed a single exercise session. However, under certain conditions, it is best to delay exercise, defer for the day, or stop your exercise program until you have visited your primary care provider. Like Fran, it is likely that during the course of your aerobic exercise program you may become ill. In Fran's case, she caught a cold, an active infection. Fran should wait until the cold is over and she feels better before returning to exercise.

Chapter 9

Why Should I Be Vigilant of Behavioral and Psychological Symptoms of Dementia?

*M*iranda, 72, was diagnosed with Alzheimer's dementia five years before she enrolled in our study. She was always happy and laughed often. She told us repeatedly that she really enjoyed the exercise program. Almost unfailingly, she asked many times, minutes apart, during an exercise session why she was in the program and who signed her up for it. From time to time, Miranda moved her hands aimlessly, wrung them, or became restless. Our exercise specialist asked Miranda if she was worried about something. One of her worries was her grandson. Miranda thought her daughter forgot to *pick him up from daycare, but we knew that he was a grown man by then.*

———————————◆———————————◆———————————

Tom, 88, was diagnosed with Alzheimer's dementia three years before he enrolled in our study. During exercise sessions, he usually started to pedal at a good speed on the cycle but then slowed down. It was not because he was unable to exercise at a higher level. When our exercise specialist reminded him to pedal faster, he did sometimes, but at other times, he slowed even further or just stopped. Putting a reminder note on his cycle did not work either. When we asked him why he would not cycle faster, he responded with "I'm 88 years old. I'm doing very well for my age." At times, he simply ignored the request to speed up, smiled at us, and started to sing "You Are My Sunshine."

———————————◆———————————◆———————————

Dan, 69, was diagnosed with Alzheimer's dementia six months before he enrolled in our study. He was very easily distracted when performing a task. His wife usually packed him spare pants and a shirt to change into after the exercise sessions because he worked up a good sweat. One day, he was taking off his shoes to change his pants when another participant asked him a question. He then held one shoe and got stuck not knowing what to do next: put the shoe back on or take the other shoe off, too. He said that he did not like "being instructed around." After the exercise sessions, he walked around collecting things—especially water bottles—from other people. By the time he was ready to leave, Dan held four or five water bottles in his arms.

———————————◆———————————◆———————————

Jennifer, 79, was diagnosed with Alzheimer's dementia four years before she enrolled in our study. She asked repetitive questions during the exercise sessions and appeared irritable. She was hostile at times and commented on her dislike of both the exercise program and our exercise specialist. Our exercise specialist always asked right away if she wanted to continue exercising. Every time, Jennifer said yes. Responding to Jennifer's questions or comments with explanations sometimes appeared to irritate her further. Despite her open remarks about disliking our program, Jennifer kept returning to the exercise sessions and was one of our top performers in the end, completing 100% of all her planned exercise sessions.

The above scenarios are based on true, but modified stories of our participants, and give you a glimpse of the variety of behavioral and psychological symptoms of dementia (BPSD). Our participants are older adults still living in the community who have mild to moderate Alzheimer's dementia at study enrollment. They participated in our exercise program for as long as 50 minutes a session (not counting warm-up and cool-down), three times a week for six months under the guidance and supervision of our exercise specialists. Understanding how to prevent and work with BPSD is one of the most important strategies to ensure exercise safety.

In this chapter, you will find out the definitions and origins of BPSD and its individual symptoms. You will learn about our Approach AD S.A.F.E.ly™ ABC-MESSS Tool to prevent and treat BPSD, which ensures ongoing exercise participation and safety for people with Alzheimer's dementia. Last, you will become familiar with the drugs used for BPSD treatment. This chapter addresses you as an exercise provider or a family caregiver.

What Are BPSD?

Reflecting on the opening scenarios, how do you think each participant's symptoms could have interfered with their exercise participation? How would you have worked with Miranda's anxiety,

Tom's resistance to exercise coaching and guidance, Dan's distraction and hoarding, and Jennifer's irritability and hostility? These symptoms used to be called by different names, such as neuropsychiatric, problematic, inappropriate, disruptive, disturbing, or noncognitive symptoms, just to name a few. It was not until 1995, when the term "behavioral and psychological signs and symptoms of dementia (BPSSD)" was coined at the Seventh International Psychogeriatric Association Congress in Sydney, Australia. After this, a shortened term, behavioral and psychological symptoms of dementia or BPSD, gained popularity and has been widely used. By definition, BPSD refers to the range of symptoms that people with Alzheimer's dementia exhibit. Psychological symptoms include depression, anxiety, psychosis (delusions and hallucinations), apathy, and disinhibition (socially and sexually inappropriate behaviors). Behavioral symptoms include agitation, aggression, and sleep disturbances.

BPSD is nearly universal in people with Alzheimer's dementia, with 90% of them having one or more symptoms during the course of their dementia. These symptoms are specifically linked to dementia due to their substantially higher rates of occurrence in people with dementia than in the general population. Among Alzheimer's triad symptoms (cognitive impairment, functional decline, and BPSD), BPSD is often the most challenging to work with and causes significant distress to family caregivers and health care providers. BPSD accounts for at least a third of the health care cost in Alzheimer's dementia due to increased caregiving time and health service use. BPSD predicts many poor health outcomes such as functional decline and nursing home placement, quickens AD progression, increases the rates of hospitalization and death, prolongs hospital stays, and induces other medical conditions.

Although the term BPSD seems to indicate that these symptoms only occur when someone has a dementia diagnosis, recent evidence suggests otherwise. BPSD can actually happen early in the course of AD. About 43% to 59% of individuals with mild cognitive impairment due to AD show at least one BPSD. BPSD in mild cognitive impairment may even predict the onset of Alzheimer's dementia. For example, late-life depression doubles the risk of Alzheimer's dementia.

There are some observable patterns of BPSD in different types of dementia. In Alzheimer's and vascular dementia, depression, anxiety, agitation (particularly irritability), and aggression occur more often. In frontotemporal dementia, it is more common to see apathy, disinhibition, and aggression.

Why Do BPSD Occur?

The origins of BPSD are complex, with many unknowns. Important progresses have been made to aid the understanding of their origins from a biophysiological perspective, such as the location of AD brain changes and the imbalance of neurotransmitters. A psychosocial perspective, such as unmet needs, behavioral triggers and reinforcement, and lowered stress tolerance, further helps the understanding. The biophysiological perspective is essential for developing drug treatments. In contrast, the psychosocial perspective is more useful for daily interactions with people who have Alzheimer's dementia, like exercise.

Biophysiological Origins of BPSD

Chapter 2 described AD brain changes as two hallmarks (amyloid plaques and neurofibrillary tangles) and several non-hallmark abnormal processes (neurodegeneration, insulin resistance and glucose hypometabolism, neuroinflammation, mitochondrial dysfunction and oxidative stress, neurochemical changes, vascular dysfunction, and infection). Individually and together, these abnormal changes cause the brain structure and circuitry to break down, leading to BPSD.

The location of AD brain changes gives rise to specific cognitive impairment and BPSD that seem to occur together but not necessarily at the same time. For example, AD brain changes affecting the prefrontal lobes may cause executive dysfunction and apathy. AD brain changes affecting the right parietal lobe may cause visuospatial deficit and hallucination. Furthermore, BPSD may be caused by the imbalance of neurotransmitters. Because different neurotransmitters perform different tasks, different BPSD arise.

Psychosocial Origins of BPSD
Unmet needs

Based on the Unmet Needs model, people with Alzheimer's dementia exhibit BPSD as a way to "communicate" that some of their needs are not being met by themselves and help is needed. As AD worsens, people with Alzheimer's dementia have increasing difficulty in communicating their needs and cannot use personal, social, and environmental resources to appropriately address their needs themselves. Even when family and health care professionals have identified an unmet need, they may not have addressed the unmet needs in a way that reflects the preferences, habits, personality, and health status of people with Alzheimer's dementia. As a result, BPSD ensues.

Common unmet needs include physical discomfort (e.g., pain, hunger, thirst, and sensory deprivation), mental discomfort (e.g., fear of danger, frustration, and abandonment), inadequate social contact (e.g., overstimulation, under-stimulation, boredom, and poor communication), environmental discomfort (e.g., overcrowding, insufficient light, and too hot or cold temperature). For example, people with Alzheimer's dementia may start to fidget because they are bored. When boredom was not addressed or was inadequately addressed, it can escalate to purposeless movements such as pacing or wandering. People who are in pain or feel cold or lonely might have repetitious vocalizations such as calling out or shouting. Unless these needs are addressed, their vocalizations may continue or even get worse.

Behavioral triggers and reinforcement

According to the Antecedent-Behavior-Consequence (ABC) model, a specific stimulus (antecedent) precedes and triggers a specific behavior, which leads to a consequence. The consequence, in turn, reinforces and strengthens the behavior. For example, Rachael needed to use the bathroom but could not find her way there due to her impaired visuospatial function. Neither could she ask for help because she has trouble expressing herself. She became agitated. When her husband noticed her agitation, he realized that she probably needed to use the bathroom since she had last been there several hours before. He took her to the bathroom, and her agitation went away.

In this case, the need to use the bathroom is the antecedent, agitation is the behavior, and her husband's taking her to the bathroom is the consequence. Because the consequence is desired, the behavior, agitation, is reinforced. The next time Rachael needs to use the bathroom, she will become agitated again because agitation prompts her husband to take her to the bathroom. Hence, a regular toileting schedule could break this cycle of reinforcement and prevent agitation.

Lowered stress tolerance

The Progressively Lowered Stress Threshold model proposes that people with dementia have a progressive decline in their abilities to receive, process, and respond to internal and environmental stressors, which is defined as the lowered stress tolerance or threshold. Examples of internal stressors include pain, hunger, fatigue; impaired ability to communicate or express needs; not being understood; feeling unwanted, lonely, scared, or unloved; and need for attention, intimacy, friendship, or purpose. External stressors may include noise overload; uncomfortable room temperature, lighting, or smell; crowding; and overstimulating, impatient, or unskilled caregivers.

Stress tolerance gets progressively lower as AD worsens over time, so a stimulus appropriate for people without Alzheimer's dementia may be stressful for people with mild Alzheimer's dementia, and a stimulus appropriate for people with mild Alzheimer's dementia might be too much for people with moderate Alzheimer's dementia, and so on. On a given day, the ability to tolerate stress in people with Alzheimer's dementia also declines with time. People with dementia become less and less able to cope with stressors and perceive their environment as more and more stressful as a day goes by.

While the Unmet Needs model, ABC model, and Progressively Lowered Stress Threshold model approach BPSD from different perspectives, they overlap and complement each other. In a given situation, one model might explain a symptom better than the others, or all three models might need to be used to best work with a situation.

What Factors Increase BPSD?

The timing, course, and severity of BPSD are highly variable across individuals. BPSD can occur intermittently and fluctuate in severity over time. A wide range of factors at the person, caregiver, and environment levels can trigger BPSD.

- Person-level factors include medical issues such as undiagnosed medical problems; infections; drug-drug interactions; inadequate treatment of symptoms such as pain;

longstanding personality traits and behavioral patterns; physical needs such as thirst, hunger, or toileting; and emotional needs such as comfort, respect, and love.

- Caregiver-level factors include high levels of stress, depression, and anxiety; low levels of health and well-being; negative communication styles such as anger, yelling, or harsh tone; false or unrealistic expectations of people with Alzheimer's dementia; misinterpretation of BPSD; and lack of social and professional support.

- Environment-level factors are composed of objects (furniture in the home and their locations); temperature (too hot or cold); noise (too noisy or quiet); lighting (not enough or too much); and social and cultural values and beliefs related to Alzheimer's dementia and care.

Despite the wide variations in BPSD, certain trends seem to exist. Women tend to have more symptoms than men. The recurrence rates of BPSD are significantly greater in people with multiple symptoms than those with just one symptom. Psychosis, depression, agitation, and aggression are linked to increased nursing home admission, but not consistently.

Another well-known feature of BPSD is sundowning, or sundown syndrome, in which BPSD occurs or worsens in the late afternoon and early evening. Sundowning contributes to poor health outcomes such as rapid cognitive decline, increased caregiver burden, and early nursing home admission. Sundowning is estimated to affect 2% to 66% of people with Alzheimer's dementia, depending on the methods used for assessing sundowning and the participants studied. AD brain changes, particularly hyperphosphorylated tau, are believed to change the melatonin level and cholinergic transmission in the brain, which impairs the circadian rhythm, leading to sundowning.

What Can I Expect of Each Symptom?

The exact BPSD that people with Alzheimer's dementia exhibits is highly variable. Each symptom of BPSD has its own unique prevalence, course, and impact. It is necessary to distinguish the terms used for the psychological symptoms from those representing medical diagnoses. For example, depression in the context of BPSD refers to the presence of depressive symptoms, whereas depression in the context of a medical diagnosis refers to a major depressive disorder or clinical depression. In other words, when people with Alzheimer's dementia are said to have depression, they do not necessarily have a diagnosis of major depressive disorder.

Depression

Depression is manifested as depressed mood and markedly diminished interest or pleasure in all, or almost all, activities. It could also show up as decreased or increased appetite; slowed thought processes; reduced physical movements (noticeable not just by the affected person); fatigue or loss of energy; feelings of worthlessness or excessive or inappropriate guilt; indecision or diminished ability to think or concentrate; and recurrent thoughts of death, suicidal ideation with or without a specific plan, and suicide attempt.

Depression is one of the most common BPSD, seen in 25% to 75% of people with Alzheimer's dementia. Each year, about 17% of people with Alzheimer's dementia develop depression, and about 40% will have depression within the next five years. Depression markedly reduces quality of life, causes rapid cognitive and functional decline, and increases the risk of death and early nursing home placement.

Depression is not merely a psychological reaction to having Alzheimer's dementia, and it seems to differ from conventional clinical depression. Conventional depression results from deficits in monoamine neurotransmitters (serotonergic or noradrenergic abnormalities) in the brain; hence, antidepressant drugs that restore these neurotransmitters are effective in treating depression. However, they generally have a poor to modest effect on depression in people with Alzheimer's dementia. Recent findings suggest that depression in people with Alzheimer's dementia arises from alterations in glutamatergic neurotransmitters.

Imaging studies linked depression to low metabolism in the left dorsolateral prefrontal region of the brain, suggesting that depression might result from AD's damage to brain regions involved in mood regulation. Nonetheless, depression might not entirely depend on AD brain changes because genetic factors such as the apolipoprotein (*APOE*) gene seem to play a role. The *APOE* 4 allele has been linked to a fourfold increase in depression in women with Alzheimer's dementia.

Anxiety

Anxiety refers to excessive fear or worry and other symptoms that make it hard to carry out daily activities and responsibilities. Fear and worry are both emotional responses. They overlap but are different. Fear is about an existing or perceived imminent threat and is often linked to "fight or flight" responses and escape behaviors. Worry is the anticipation of a future threat and is often linked to cautious or avoidant behaviors. Other symptoms of anxiety include: 1) restlessness or edginess (feeling keyed up or on edge); 2) fatigue (becoming easily fatigued or more fatigued than usual); 3) difficulty concentrating or the mind going blank; 4) irritability that others may or may not perceive; 5) muscle tension (increased muscle aches or soreness); and 6) sleep disturbances (difficulty falling or staying asleep, restlessness at night, or unsatisfying sleep).

Anxiety is seen in 48% to 52% of people with Alzheimer's dementia and is most apparent in the mild stage. In the later stages of Alzheimer's dementia, anxiety can be hard to recognize. Social disengagement or withdrawal from once pleasurable activities, typical in depression, may also reflect anxiety. Shadowing (following family members), crying, calling out repeatedly, and having angry outbursts can also be signs of anxiety. Imaging studies have shown that higher amyloid burden, measured by positron emission tomography, is linked to increased anxiety over time in older adults with normal cognition.

Psychosis

Psychosis is the "gross impairment in reality testing" or "loss of ego boundaries" that interferes with a person's ability to carry out daily activities. Psychosis includes delusion and hallucination. Delusion is characterized by a paranoid or fixed false or incorrect belief. For example, people with Alzheimer's dementia may think that someone is harming them, a spouse is being unfaithful, or someone is stealing from them. Hallucination is a sensory perception in the absence of a corresponding stimulus, such as seeing or hearing things that are not there. The affected person may not have the ability to recognize that the stimulus is not real.

Psychosis is seen in 20% of people with Alzheimer's dementia. Delusion by itself occurs in 13% to 55% of people with Alzheimer's dementia, with paranoid delusion being the most common. Hallucination is seen in about 11% of people with Alzheimer's dementia, with visual hallucination being more common than an auditory hallucination. Psychosis is the least common but most serious symptom in mild Alzheimer's dementia. Psychosis is linked to greater initial cognitive dysfunction, faster cognitive decline, physical aggression, early nursing home admission, and high rate of death.

Psychosis has been related to the severity of AD-associated neurodegeneration. People with Alzheimer's dementia and psychosis have a greater accumulation of abnormal tau and amyloid. Psychosis has also been associated with serotonin receptor abnormality and low metabolism in the frontal lobes, particularly the orbitofrontal and lateral frontal regions. Delusion is linked to a reduced metabolic activity in the right lateral frontal cortex, orbitofrontal cortex, and bilateral temporal cortex; and hallucination to atrophy of the parietal lobe. Having *APOE* allele 4 also seems to increase the risk of psychosis.

Apathy

Apathy is a cluster of motivational deficits expressed by a lack of feeling, emotion, interest, or concern. Apathy is reportedly the most common BPSD in Alzheimer's dementia, followed by depression, irritability, and agitation. Apathy is seen in 72% to 88% of people with Alzheimer's dementia. Apathy and depression often co-exist, with about 23% to 32% of people with Alzheimer's dementia having both, suggesting that apathy and depression may share a common origin.

Apathy is specifically correlated with low metabolism in the left orbitofrontal lobe. Positron emission tomography scans show that people with Alzheimer's dementia and apathy have more amyloid plaques in the bilateral frontal cortex than people with Alzheimer's dementia but no apathy. However, cortical thinning in the temporal cortex has also been linked to more severe apathy over time.

Disinhibition

Disinhibition refers to undue familiarity and impulsive comments and actions shown by a lack of restraint, such as disregard of social norms and impulsivity. Disinhibition is seen in 7% to 36% of people with Alzheimer's dementia who display socially inappropriate behaviors (e.g., statements inappropriate in a social interaction).

Inappropriate sexual behaviors are physical or verbal acts with a sexual meaning or intent, or persistent, uninhibited sexual behaviors directed at oneself or others. Inappropriate sexual behaviors have an estimated prevalence of 2% to 30%. They can be difficult to manage, leading to significant strain and distress for families and health care professionals. Both disinhibition and aggression have major effects on social functioning. Imaging studies have shown that the prefrontal cortex, particularly the orbitofrontal area, plays a critical role in regulating the inhibition and disinhibition circuitry.

Agitation

Agitation is a broad category of symptoms that includes restlessness, pacing, arguing, disruptive vocalizations, and resistance to care (e.g., rejecting other people's assistance in activities such as bathing, dressing, and grooming). Agitation is one of the most common BPSD, seen in 24% to 60% of people with Alzheimer's dementia. Irritability is seen in 42% to 60% of people with Alzheimer's dementia and is exhibited as an excessive response to stimuli.

Wandering may be considered as extreme agitation. Wandering is seen in 39% to 57% of people with Alzheimer's disease and consists of moving about without a definite destination or purpose. However, wandering and resistance to care are believed to not fall neatly into either the psychological or behavioral symptom category of BPSD.

Agitation is most often seen in men who are in the advanced stages of Alzheimer's dementia. Agitation contributes to poor health outcomes, such as cognitive decline, loss of independence, emotional distress, caregiver burden, nursing home admission, death, excessive psychomotor activity, and other BPSD such as aggression, irritability, and disinhibition.

Agitation seems to arise from specific neurochemical changes in the brain, such as an imbalance of serotonin in the frontal lobe. Imaging studies have linked agitation to greater atrophy in a number of regions in the frontal, cingulate, temporal, amygdala, and hippocampal cortices. The *APOE* allele 4 is also associated with aggression.

Aggression

Aggression is a hostile, forceful behavior or disposition directed at a person or the environment. Aggression can be classified as physical (directed at others such as hitting, kicking or biting or at oneself such as pacing or inappropriately handling objects) or verbal (directed at others such as cursing or at oneself such as repetition of words or sentences). Aggression, which is seen in 6% to 66% of people with Alzheimer's dementia, affects the quality of life, contributes to cognitive decline and loss of independence, and is a common cause of nursing home admission.

Aggression is the most common in men and in the advanced stages of Alzheimer's dementia. Psychosis and aggression are highly correlated. Delusion is among the strongest predictors of aggression, which suggests that delusion may drive the onset of aggression.

Neurotransmitter dysfunction, such as serotonin, norepinephrine, and N-acetyl aspartate-to-creatinine ratio, has been implicated in aggression. Aggression has been linked to hippocampal neurofibrillary tangles, reduced metabolism in the temporal lobe, and atrophy in many brain regions such as the frontal cortex, amygdala, and hippocampus.

Sleep Disturbances

Sleep disturbances refer to sleep-related changes such as poor sleep quality and long durations of sleep (more than eight hours). Sleep disturbances become more common with age and negatively affect memory and other cognitive function. AD brain changes aggravate sleep disturbances by altering the sleep-wake or circadian rhythm. About 70% of people with Alzheimer's dementia have sleep disturbances, most often nighttime awakenings and low sleep efficiency (the proportion of time in sleep to time spent in bed).

AD brain changes affect areas of the brain (e.g., the suprachiasmatic nuclei and lateral hypothalamic area) that play a key role in regulating sleep. Inadequate sleep, such as decreased slow-wave sleep, impairs amyloid and tau clearance from the cerebral interstitial fluid.

In summary, the presence, timing, and severity of each symptom vary greatly across people with Alzheimer's dementia and over the course of AD. Table 9.1 provides a summary of the BPSD.

How Can BPSD Be Treated?

The good news is that BPSD can be effectively prevented, reduced, and managed. Vigilance about BPSD is required when working with people with Alzheimer's dementia to ensure that the triggers for BPSD are identified and managed. Like a detective's work, the chance of finding the "criminal" (trigger for BPSD) is increased when a systematic approach is taken to identify triggers at the person, caregiver, and environment levels. It is helpful to think about the trigger as an unmet need, antecedent, or stimulus beyond the threshold of stress tolerance. If a trigger can be identified, specific strategies to prevent and treat BPSD, described below, can be used. If a trigger cannot be identified, a trial-and-error approach must be taken to identify the right strategy.

BPSD Prevention and Treatment

BPSD prevention and treatment rely on non-drug interventions and person-centered care. Non-drug interventions, or psychosocial, behavioral, or nonpharmacologic interventions, are the first-line or initial treatments for BPSD, endorsed by many professional organizations such as the American Geriatrics Society, the American Psychiatric Association, and the American Association for Geriatric Psychiatry. The effectiveness of some of these

Table 9.1. Definition and Prevalence of Behavioral and Psychological Symptoms of Dementia

Symptoms	Definition	Prevalence
Aggression	Behavior or disposition that is hostile, forceful, and attacking	6%–66%
Agitation	Excitement and restlessness	24%–60%
Anxiety	Pacing back and forth, rumination, and somatic complaints	48%–52%
Apathy	A lack of feeling, emotion, interest, or concern	72%–88%
Delusion	Paranoid beliefs (e.g., people are stealing things)	13%–55%
Depression	Sadness and loss of interest in usual activities, guilt, and hopelessness	25%–75%
Disinhibition	Impulsivity and disregard of social norms	7%–36%
Hallucinations	Visual or auditory (see or hear things that are not there)	~11%
Irritability	Excessive response to stimuli	42%–60%
Psychosis	Elevated or irritable mood, hyperactivity, intrusiveness, impulsivity, and reduced sleep, and pressured speech	~20%
Sleep disturbances	Sleep-related changes such as poor sleep quality and long	~70%

interventions have been inconsistent or remain to be established because of variations in the study participants, measures of BPSD, specific symptoms studied, and numbers of study participants. Non-drug interventions also reduce inappropriate medication use. Currently, the evidence is the strongest for caregiver interventions such as problem-solving to identify triggers for BPSD, enhance communications with people affected by AD, and change the culture and attitudes of family and health care professionals about BPSD.

The ABC-MESSS Tool

Built on the evidence of non-drug interventions, our Approach AD S.A.F.E.ly™ ABC-MESSS Tool is used for BPSD prevention and treatment. ABC-MESSS is the acronym of AD education; Behavioral modification; Cognition- and emotion-oriented interventions; Medical and nursing interventions; Environmental design; Social interaction; Structured activities; and Sensory enhancement or relaxation.

- AD education: Education about AD is absolutely critical for empowering people with Alzheimer's dementia and their family caregivers to understand AD and seek help, and for exercise providers to safely screen and supervise exercise participation for people with Alzheimer's dementia. In our studies, we educate our study staff on AD clinical course, symptoms, abnormal brain processes, risk and protective factors, effects of aerobic exercise on AD abnormal processes, and person-centered care and communication skills, as covered in previous chapters.

- Behavioral modification: We explain the unacceptable nature of some behaviors that can cause substantial stress to others such as derogatory sexual remarks. We reinforce desirable behaviors through social interaction. We also recognize and remove a stimulus that causes BPSD such as a contentious topic among our study participants.

- Cognition- and emotion-oriented interventions: We use validation to help our study participants express their emotions, and reminiscence to get to know our participants better over time.
- Medical and nursing interventions: We work with our participants and their families to make sure that our participants wear appropriate sensory aids such as reading glasses and hearing aids; seek medical evaluation as needed; and have symptoms such as pain properly managed.
- Environmental design: We can do little to change the physical environment because our exercise program is delivered at the facilities of our community partners. However, we can control certain aspects of the social and cultural environment to make it as friendly as possible to our participants. If you are able to modify a physical environment, consider including natural sounds, such as recorded music, bird chirps, babbling brooks, and ocean waves; simulated home environment for people with Alzheimer's dementia living in senior facilities; visual contrast using colors; and avoidance of overstimulation such as turning off the TV.
- Social interaction: Social interaction is important to our participants and is one of the motivators to keep them engaged in our exercise program. In our recent study, the Efficacy and Mechanisms of Combined Aerobic Exercise and Cognitive Training (ACT) in MCI or the ACT Trial, we had to build in a 10-minute socialization time to our study sessions to meet our participants' needs to socialize after a session. Other researchers have shown that social

interaction can occur as one-on-one or in a group format, simulated using technology, and assisted by pet therapy.

- Structured activities: Establishing a daily routine for exercise has been perceived as very beneficial by family caregivers in our studies. A daily routine that meets the needs of each person with Alzheimer's dementia also helps reduce stress. Examples of other routine activities include cognitive and sensory-stimulating activities; arts; and outdoor or nature walks.

- Sensory enhancement or relaxation: We could not use these techniques much as they could compromise the rigor of our study designs, but they can be easily used by family caregivers and health care professionals to prevent or mitigate BPSD. They include massage or therapeutic touch; music (listening to music, playing instruments, singing, and dancing); white noise; visual sensory stimulation (videos of family members talking to people with Alzheimer's dementia; light therapy); and multisensory stimulations using hearing, touch, and smell (aromatherapy, cooking groups, and building activities).

In summary, our Approach AD S.A.F.E.ly™ ABC-MESSS Tool supports the use of a combination of interventions to prevent and treat BPSD to ensure exercise engagement and safety for people with Alzheimer's dementia. Not all interventions will work for each person, and the combination of interventions used may change over time. Some interventions, such as music, may be used relatively easily, while others, such as AD education, require invested time, effort, and planning. It is also important to note that an intervention that worked previously might not work in the future, and vice versa. Hence, our ABC-MESSS Tool needs to be personalized as described below.

Personalizing the ABC-MESSS Tool

Person-centered care is essential to work with BPSD because the timing and severity of BPSD vary greatly across individuals. It is important to invest the time to get to know people with Alzheimer's dementia and their family and social contexts to guide intervention selection.

Different BPSD respond to different interventions. One-on-one interaction that is effective for addressing agitation due to boredom is not useful for hallucination. The effectiveness of an ABC-MESSS intervention depends on many factors such as medical, psychosocial, and environmental conditions; lifelong habits; personality before Alzheimer's dementia; family and social relationships; and cultural background and values. Studies have found that interventions mapped to previous habits, hobbies, and personality are effective at reducing BPSD.

If depression arises from emotional responses to having Alzheimer's dementia, such as a feeling of being useless and loss of independence, focus on the accomplishments and new or upcoming activities rather than the past activities that the person can no longer participate in. To address apathy, it is important to highlight accomplishments, provide rewards, praise efforts, and make goals attainable.

When disinhibition appears, it is useful to gently remind the person that he or she is in a public place and that others may be offended by his or her words or actions. Strategies that help minimize repetitive questioning are to explain the situation before or as it arises and to divert the conversation to a new topic that the person with Alzheimer's dementia knows. Patience and answering each question fully, as if it were the first time the question has been asked, is helpful. Wandering could be harmless unless the person becomes lost or the calories burned exceed food intake and cause weight loss or falls.

BPSD that occurs suddenly and rapidly worsens could indicate a medical condition such as drug toxicity or infection. A health care professional should assess these symptoms as soon as possible.

Drug Treatment for BPSD

A drug may be considered if BPSD shows no or minimal improvement from non-drug interventions, the person has severe behavioral symptoms, or behavioral symptoms have psychotic features that present a danger to the person or other people.

However, no drugs are approved by the U.S. Food and Drug Administration for managing BPSD. Health care professionals have to resort to the off-label use of antipsychotics, sedatives or hypnotics, anxiolytics, or antidepressants. Their effectiveness for BPSD is unknown because drug trials have shown mixed effects. Most drugs not only have limited effects and lack long-term benefits for BPSD, but they can also cause serious side effects and death.

Neuroleptics and other antipsychotics are the most common drugs used to treat agitation and aggression but have only modest effectiveness. When used long term, they significantly increase the risk of side effects such as serious cerebrovascular events, metabolic syndrome, and increased risk for death. Even well-targeted drugs (e.g., melatonin to reduce agitation) have shown inconclusive and conflicting results. As a result, efforts to limit the use of conventional and atypical antipsychotics in Alzheimer's dementia are underway in the United States and around the world. Due to their limited effectiveness and side effects, antipsychotic drugs now carry a warning of the increased risk for death from any causes in people with dementia.

Before starting a drug, people with Alzheimer's dementia and their family members need to discuss a drug exit plan with the health care providers, so the providers can regularly evaluate if the drug dose can be reduced, with the goal of eventually stopping the drug. Some indications for stopping include the lack of effectiveness, intolerable side effects, and stabilized symptoms.

It is important to point out that designating non-drug interventions, as the first-line treatment for BPSD does not preclude the use of drugs if needed. Non-drug interventions are often effective at first but may stop working later. For some people, drugs may be the only option. On the other hand, stabilized symptoms do not necessarily mean that there are no unmet needs or antecedents for BPSD. In this case, a drug may mask or disguise the unmet needs that are still there, which could limit the ability of family caregivers and health care professionals to provide needed care to people with Alzheimer's dementia.

Key Messages

- BPSD occur in most people with Alzheimer's dementia and include depression, anxiety, psychosis (delusion and hallucination), apathy, disinhibition, agitation, aggression, and sleep disturbances.
- The presence, timing, and severity of each symptom vary greatly across people with Alzheimer's dementia and over the course of AD. BPSD tends to occur in the late afternoon or early evening, a phenomenon called sundowning.
- BPSD are likely the result of damage to certain areas of the brain and neurotransmitter imbalance caused by AD brain changes.
- BPSD represents an unmet need, reinforcement of a behavioral response to an antecedent, or decreased stress tolerance.
- BPSD affects exercise participation and safety and can be prevented and managed using our Approach AD S.A.F.E.ly™ ABC-MESSS Tool.

- ABC-MESSS represents <u>A</u>D education; <u>B</u>ehavioral modification; <u>C</u>ognition- and emotion-oriented interventions; <u>M</u>edical and nursing interventions; <u>E</u>nvironmental design; <u>S</u>ocial interaction; <u>S</u>tructured activities; and <u>S</u>ensory enhancement or relaxation.
- Our Approach AD S.A.F.E.ly™ protocol supports the use of a combination of the ABC-MESSS interventions in a personalized fashion to prevent and treat BPSD to ensure exercise engagement and safety for people with Alzheimer's dementia.
- Drugs should be used as the last resort for BPSD due to their limited effectiveness and high likelihood of side effects.

The Beginning Scenarios

Now, let us reflect on the cases at the beginning of this chapter. How would you work with Miranda's repetitive questioning and anxiety? Our exercise specialist answered each question as if it were asked for the very first time. Miranda was easily satisfied with the answers. She laughed, made a joke, carried on, and asked the same question again a few minutes later. When Miranda showed signs of anxiety, our exercise specialist asked Miranda if she would feel better if she (the exercise specialist) called Miranda's daughter to confirm. Miranda became calm within minutes of the call.

What about Tom's resistance to exercising harder when he was fully capable of it? Our exercise specialist wrote the range of speed she wanted him to pedal on a sticky note and placed it next to his cycle's speed display. When it was time to increase his speed, our exercise specialist asked him to pedal faster and replaced the note with a new one. Another strategy that worked sometimes was when our exercise specialist pedaled next to him and suggested that they kept pace.

How would you have worked with Dan's distraction and hoarding symptoms? Our exercise specialist addressed his distraction by breaking down a multistep task to one step at a time, but you may recall that Dan said that he did not like "being instructed around." Our exercise specialist spoke to his wife, who said that Dan really respected authority, so our exercise specialist said, "I know you do not like to be told, but it is one of the rules I need to follow when we work together." We suspected that his hoarding of water bottles was an extension of his former occupation as a sports coach. Our exercise specialist kept an eye on where he got the bottles and said, "Thank you for helping clean. I can take the bottles now and put them in the right place."

Would you feel hurt if you were exercising with Jennifer and she told you often that she did not like you? Our exercise specialist knew not to take Jennifer's comments about disliking her personally. When Jennifer appeared irritated by the responses to her questions, it worked to change the topic of conversation or temporarily disengage from the conversation.

Chapter 10

How Do I Manage Alzheimer's Symptoms During Exercise?

J oan suddenly woke with the horrible feeling that she was late! She hated being late or making others wait for her. She looked out the window and, sure enough, the university car to take her to her exercise session was already outside waiting for her. She shot out of bed and got dressed, ignoring her husband who told her that the university car was not there and that it was 2 a.m. However, she knew her husband was wrong. She finished getting dressed, got her bag and water, and went outside. Only then did she realize it was not the university car; it was a neighbor's car, and it was, indeed, 2 a.m. She went back inside and slept until 7 a.m. when her alarm was set to ring.

The Alzheimer's Rx: Aerobic Exercise

David and Alex had been exercising in the same sessions for several weeks. Alex had a great sense of humor and loved to tell jokes. David thought Alex was funny and liked his jokes. However, one day, David was not in a very good mood. Alex's jokes were starting to irritate him, so he just ignored Alex. Alex was not getting the normal response from David. Usually, David laughed at his jokes and would often respond with a witty retort. Alex decided that his jokes needed to be funnier to make David laugh. Alex's jokes got more and more outlandish, but David kept ignoring him. David could feel his patience wearing thin; he was already in a bad mood, and Alex was getting crude and annoying. Then Alex told a joke that offended David, who snapped, reached over, and punched Alex! That would get him to stop!

Catherine's exercise session was over. Julie, our student driver, took her home. When they arrived at Catherine's house, Julie pulled into her driveway, and Catherine hopped out. She told Julie she was going around the house to the back door. Julie asked her to wave through the front window once she got inside so she knew it was OK to leave. Catherine said sure; she had done this routine before. Catherine went around to the back door but could not figure out how to open it. She rummaged through her bag. She had a phone, water bottle, notebook, and a bunch of other stuff, but nothing looked like it would help. After searching for a few minutes, Catherine looked up to see Julie walking towards her. Julie asked Catherine if she wanted her to look through the bag. Catherine gladly handed it over. Julie searched for a few moments and then pulled out a key ring. Julie said, "I found it deep down in the corner!" Julie tried the keys in the back door, but none of them worked, so they walked to the front door, where a key unlocked it. Catherine was so relieved that Julie was there to help her.

———————•————————————•———————

Jack had been attending our exercise sessions for a few weeks and really loved his time with the study. He was able to talk to other people about the news, especially Prince, who had just passed away. One day, Jack returned home from his exercise session to find that his belongings were not where he had left them in his bedroom. Jack lived in a group home. He thought that one of the residents had gone into his room and rearranged his things. Two days later, when our driver arrived to pick him up for exercise, Jack refused to come, saying that he was not going to let someone rummage through his belongings while he was gone. Despite assurance from the group home staff and study staff, who offered different solutions to make sure no one touched his belongings, he refused to attend the study from that day forward.

The above scenarios are true but modified stories from our FIT-AD™ Trial, in which older adults with mild-to-moderate Alzheimer's dementia exercised three days a week for six months. Each exercise session lasted 30 minutes in the beginning and progressed to 60 minutes over time. We provided transportation for the participants between home and gym. Can you identify the Alzheimer's symptoms in each case that may have affected exercise participation?

In this chapter, you will gain knowledge of our Approach AD S.A.F.E.ly™ HAPI Tool to get to know people with Alzheimer's dementia and their family and social contexts. Then you will read real-life stories from our studies which illustrate how our exercise specialist has responded to cognitive, functional, behavioral and psychological symptoms of dementia (BPSD) during exercise sessions using our ABC-MESSS Tool introduced in Chapter 9. This chapter is written primarily from our exercise specialist's perspectives and addresses you as an exercise provider whose clients are people with Alzheimer's dementia. You can also use our HAPI and ABC-MESSS Tools for working with Alzheimer's symptoms outside of exercise.

What Is the HAPI Tool?

If you have faithfully read the previous chapters, then you probably recognize the importance of getting to know your clients, which you can achieve using our Approach AD S.A.F.E.ly™ HAPI Tool. HAPI, which is pronounced as "happy," stands for: Have the right attitude; Ask the family caregiver, Pick out a routine that works for everyone; and Initiate on day one.

Have the Right Attitude

Chapter 6 has explained the importance of nonverbal communication because your clients have difficulty communicating. Your attitude will often be mirrored by your clients.

In our studies, if I greeted our participants with a smile and was excited to see them, they often greeted me the same way. It made them feel good that someone (me) was excited to see and spend time with them. If I had a busy day with many sessions and appeared stressed, they picked up on it and did not have as much fun. I made it a point to be cheerful and smile when greeting them. There were many days when I was stressed out or had a long day of responding to symptoms of Alzheimer's disease (AD), but when someone walked in the door, I smiled.

Ask the Family Caregiver

Ask the family caregiver the same questions you asked your client, so you can have a better understanding of your client and develop topics of conversation for the first exercise session. It is also important to find out from the family caregivers which topics to avoid in conversations, AD symptoms exhibited by your clients, strategies that caregivers have found useful, and their perception of your client's level of awareness of AD.

In our studies, over time, I have learned more and more about each participant, similarly to how normal friendships develop. This allowed me to really personalize time with each participant. I would ask how their family members were doing, how an event went, or how projects at home were going. The participants often reciprocated and would ask me about my family and events in my life. This made me seem more like a friend than someone who was paid to work with them. In the end, I truly did consider the participants my friends.

Pick out a Routine that Works for Everyone

Another way to learn about your clients is to observe their habits and behaviors. Once you know your clients, you will also be able to place them in the same exercise sessions. Group exercise provides additional rapport and enjoyment for your clients if you can develop a routine that works for everyone. When you have multiple clients in one session, it is a good idea to start them about 1.5 to 2 minutes apart so you have enough time to assess each client's exercise responses without being rushed.

In our FIT-AD™ Trial, I learned who needed to use the bathroom or stop to get water and would want to chat first, as well as how much time these activities would take before and after each session. I also learned where each person kept his or her belongings (e.g., pockets for house keys, exercise logbook, and phone).

Here is an example of an exercise session routine I picked out for Ernie and Mike to exercise together:

9:30 a.m.　Ernie and Mike arrive at the YMCA.

9:40 a.m.　Take off their coats and set down their belongings.

9:45 a.m.　Use the bathroom. Mike takes about twice as long as Ernie to do this.

9:50 a.m.   Ernie returns from the bathroom, puts on heart rate monitor, and sits on cycle.

9:55 a.m.   Mike returns from the bathroom, puts on heart rate monitor, and sits on cycle.

10 a.m.   Record Ernie's resting heart rate. Turn on the cycle.

10:03 a.m.   Ernie begins warm-up. Record Mike's resting heart rate and blood pressure and turn on the cycle.

10:05 a.m.   Mike begins warm-up.

10:08 a.m.   Ernie reaches the target heart rate range and begins 50 minutes of cycling at that range.

10:10 a.m.   Mike reaches his target heart rate range and begins 50 minutes of cycling at that range.

10:58 a.m.   Ernie begins cool down.

11:00 a.m.   Mike begins cool down.

11:03 a.m.   Ernie finishes cycling and goes to the bathroom.

11:05 a.m.   Mike finishes cycling and goes to the bathroom. Ernie returns from the bathroom.

11:10 a.m.   Take Ernie's post-exercise heart rate and write his exercise summary in his notebook.

11:15 a.m.   Mike returns from the bathroom. Write his exercise summary in his notebook while he rests.

11:20 a.m.   Take Mike's post-exercise heart rate.

11:25 a.m.   Mike and Ernie gather their belongings and put on coats.

11:30 a.m.   Mike and Ernie leave for the day.

As you can see, this session takes about two hours from the time they arrive to the time they leave. Exercise sessions like this (5-minute warm-up, 50-minute cycling at target intensity, and 5-minute cool-down) usually take 1.25 to 1.5 hours, but Mike and Ernie need extra time. Ernie needs about 10 minutes per bathroom break. After a few weeks, I had this routine down to the minute, and it worked perfectly for both of them. It considers the time they needed before and after the session to use the bathroom. Not listed in the routine was the socialization during the session, which helped us know each other and strengthen our rapport. Although I did not rush them, we were efficient with time by getting Ernie on the cycle while Mike was still in the bathroom, then getting Mike on the cycle as soon as he was done. This cut down on the time Ernie had to wait for Mike.

Initiate on Day One

From the first day, make a conscious effort to get to know your clients and their family and social contexts. Ask your clients what they like to be called, likes, dislikes, hobbies, previous occupations, communication preferences, and perceptions of AD symptoms and their effects on their lives.

In our studies, we train our study staff to make sure they know the importance of the initial encounter with our potential participants. We spent many hours practicing the screening process, which really helped us to get to know the participants.

How Do I Respond to Cognitive Symptoms?

During exercise sessions, I have observed a few common cognitive symptoms: repetitive questioning, memory impairment, and impaired judgment. AD education and cognition- and emotion-oriented interventions from our ABC-MESSS Tool are particularly useful for understanding and addressing these symptoms.

Repetitive Questioning

Repetitive questioning can indicate memory impairment, anxiety, or both. One participant, Arthur, became anxious if our driver did not pull into his driveway at exactly the pickup time. His wife, Marcia, would try to reassure him that the university car was coming to pick him up, but it was no use. Arthur would repeatedly ask his wife, "Are they coming? Are they coming? Is it canceled? Are they coming?" without end until the car arrived. If I called to let them know of a major delay on the road (uncommon, but it happened from time to time), Marcia would drive Arthur to the YMCA herself to stop the repetitive questioning.

The questioning did not stop once Arthur arrived at the YMCA. He would repeatedly say, "I am ready to go. I am ready to go. Are you ready to start? I am ready to go." The exercise room we used has floor-to-ceiling windows with a clear view of all vehicles coming and going in the parking lot, which proved problematic for Arthur. Once he started his exercise session, Arthur watched the parking lot and, for each car that drove by, would repeatedly ask, "Is that my car? Is that my car? Is that my car?" to which I replied that it was not his car. If he was not on that line of questioning, he would repeatedly say, "I am ready to go home. I am ready to go home. I am ready to go home and take a nap. I am ready to go home." Sometimes, he changed it a little and told me what was for lunch before the nap, which, without fail, was a cheese sandwich.

Whenever possible, I would use a different exercise room. If that was not possible, I positioned Arthur with his back to the windows. Another strategy was to count aloud ("1, 2, 3 ...."). Arthur would voluntarily join in the counting, which distracted him from the repetitive questioning. However, I was careful not to let him get overexcited because he sometimes would grab the hand of the participant next to him and swing his arms while counting. I wanted to avoid this because it could have caused him or the other participant to go off balance and fall.

Honestly, the repetitive questioning or statements can be quite difficult to work with. If I did not interrupt Arthur or distract him, he could go straight without a break in the repetition (likely, the entire 50 minutes). I contacted Marcia and their daughter for tips to break the repetition, and they said that Arthur and Marcia had traveled quite extensively and continued to travel. Also, Marcia was a good photographer, and they had many albums of pictures from their travels. I learned that if I asked him about the travels or photographs, it gave us a brief reprieve from the repetition. Distraction would work for a few minutes at most, but it was short-lived if a car drove by. Ultimately, I had to practice patience and live in his reality. Although he had already asked several times if his car was there, I answered as if it were the first time. Despite his repetitive questioning, Arthur was a wonderful person and quite enjoyable to work with.

Memory Impairment

Memory impairment presents a challenge when I need to ascertain certain aspects of the participants' medical conditions. For example, they may not be able to recall if they felt any discomfort after the last exercise session, whether they had taken their medications, and if they had done any exercise since the previous session.

One strategy I used was to confirm their answers with family caregivers. If the caregiver was not there, I would text or call to ask. If the caregiver was there, he or she could discreetly answer without the participant seeing. This scenario usually unfolded without consequence. However, some people with Alzheimer's dementia may not positively perceive the need to contact caregivers.

Once, a participant, Laura, was unsure if she had taken her medications that morning. I glanced at her sister, Julia, for an indication of yes or no. Laura saw my eyes slide to Julia and became furious that I was looking at Julia rather than her. In my experience, caregivers often gave me a silent head nod or shake, unseen by the participant, to indicate whether medications had been taken. I could then say something like, "Well, you are a pretty routine guy, so I doubt you missed your meds this morning" or "Hmm, well, since you are not sure, for now, I will mark down that you did not take them" in order to not indicate that the caregiver had answered me. However, this time, Laura caught me. I immediately apologized and was able to calm her. I also distracted her by changing the subject to something more fun than medications, and she quickly forgot about the entire situation. We had a very pleasant visit then.

Impaired Judgment

The most important implication of impaired judgment is that I do not know whether I can rely on the subjective rating of perceived exertion during exercise. In general, most participants could rate their exercise levels properly, but some could not grasp the concept of the rating scale. Some thought they were supposed to rate how strenuously they *wanted* to exercise rather than how strenuously they *were currently* exercising. Some wanted to impress me by rating the exercise as easier than it really was, while others rated their aches and pains while cycling.

We developed several strategies to increase the accuracy of the ratings. First, I explained how to use the scale. If that did not work, I would simplify the scale and ask if the exercise felt "easy, medium, hard, or somewhere in between" (We relate easy to an 11, medium to 13, and hard to 15). This strategy worked for some people. For participants who tried to impress me, I relied on other means to gauge exertion, such as the talk test. I always observed heart rate, sweating, labored breathing, and skin color to further assess exertion.

For those who used the scale to rate aches or pains such as "My left knee feels stiff today, so a 14," I clarified what he or she should have been rating. I validated their rating by saying something like "OK, I have that written down. Now, if you were to rate how your legs and lungs are feeling, what would you say?" Using validation, I acknowledged that they had some stiffness but also directed them to rate their exertion level. Using these strategies, I was able to get a rating of some sort from everyone who had difficulty due to impaired judgment.

How Do I Work with Functional Symptoms?

Participants with functional symptoms needed the most help from me. Common functional symptoms during exercise are cycle use, walking and balance, toileting, and hydration. AD education and structured activities from our ABC-MESSS Tool are useful for working with these symptoms.

Cycle Use

Getting their feet into the cycle pedals turned out to be difficult for our participants due to decreased depth perception and coordination. They often put their feet in the pedals with the pedals upside down. To assist, I positioned myself in front of the cycle, facing the participant. I pulled the pedal towards myself (away from the participant) until it was at a mid-to-low height, which allowed more space between the participant's body and the pedal to maneuver the foot. Then, I guided the feet into each pedal. If someone was prone to letting his or her feet slip out during cycling, I used a small bungee cord to wrap around the back of his or her foot and hold it in place while cycling.

Walking and Balance

AD brain changes affect postural control and gait stability, causing balance and walking issues. When I noticed a change in balance and walking abilities, I activated a plan to ensure the participant's safety.

For people who have a known fall risk, I used a gait belt. A gait belt is a device to help someone with fall risk safely move. It is about three inches wide and worn around the waist over clothes. I stood to the back and side of the participant and held onto the belt in back. Hand positioning is important. I used an underhand grip with the palm of the hand facing out. While walking, I was "hip to hip" with the participant. That way, I was there to steady the person if he or she started to lose balance.

For others who were not a fall risk but were just a little "wobbly," I did not use the gait belt. Rather, I just took extra care during certain situations such as walking over a curb or the gap in an elevator, maneuvering into a chair, and getting on and off the cycle. I walked next to the participant and offered an arm or hand, helped them on and off the cycle, helped them move a chair, ensured they were lined up with the chair before sitting, and gave verbal cues: "We are going to step over this curb," "Take one more step to your left before sitting," and "Let us pull the chair out a bit more before trying to sit."

Toileting

I structured the session flow by reminding the participants to use the bathroom before starting exercise and plan for mid-session bathroom breaks. Part of getting to know your clients is whether they can navigate to the bathroom and back without getting lost and what to do when two or more participants were in an exercise session.

If it was the first time the participants needed to use the bathroom, I asked if they knew the way, pointed them in the right direction, and let them go on their own. I positioned myself so I could watch them all the way into the bathroom from the cycles. If they went into the wrong hallway, I went over and said something like, "Actually, there is a closer bathroom right over here!" This language worked really well because I did not point out that they went the wrong way, only that there was a closer option. I then waited at the bathroom and returned to the cycle with them. In the subsequent sessions, I followed the same routine a few times. If, after a few times, they were not able to navigate on their own, I knew that I needed to walk them over and back each time. To show respect, I would say something like, "I'll walk over with you. I want a drink from the water fountain anyway!" This way, it seemed as though we both needed to go. If I was able to keep the conversation flowing, the participant would not even notice that I was escorting him or her to and from the bathroom.

It is important to give people a couple of chances on their own to promote as much independence as possible. In addition, some participants are able to learn the navigation and location with little guidance. Many participants navigated safely to and from the bathroom on their own for the first time.

If I had more than one participant in an exercise session and I needed to escort one, I would let the others know that I was going to the bathroom and would be right back. I often made a joke, saying, "Keep pedaling! I will know if you stop!" which they generally thought was funny and would reply with a witty retort.

Hydration

Hydration is often a problem and has to be structured into each exercise session because many participants avoid drinking water due to frequent urination or prefer to drink other liquids that are not hydrating. In our studies, we gave each participant a water bottle to bring to the sessions. Part of the conversation during exercise was about the best things for them to drink before, during, and after exercise. I also reminded them to drink at regular intervals during exercise and alert the caregivers to encourage water drinking at home. For participants who avoid drinking water because they have to use the bathroom, I encouraged small sips of water and reassured them that bathroom breaks were completely fine.

How Do I Work with BPSD?

Chapter 9 described our ABC-MESSS Tool, and I will bring this tool alive in this section for working with BPSD. I tailor the tool to

226

each participant based on my knowledge of the person. A trial-and-error period is often needed. Some symptoms are very easy to manage, while others take much more creativity and planning. Sometimes, BPSD can be triggered by something related to exercise (e.g., putting on the heart rate monitor) or home (e.g., difficult family relationships). At other times, the participants might just have a bad day.

Anxiety

Some participants were anxious about transportation to exercise sessions, although we coordinated and provided it for them. They could become anxious if our driver was not at their homes on the dot, or call multiple times the day before or the day of exercise to ensure they had the right days or knew who would pick them up and take them home. Most often, they asked me if their spouses knew what time to come and get them or if the driver knew their home address. These anxieties were not at the same level as Arthur's anxiety described earlier, although they often asked more than once. They were quite easily calmed when their questions were answered and almost all responded by saying, "Oh, that is right!" It is very important not to respond with "Do you remember?" or "I just told you."

A few participants called me multiple times a week, sometimes three or four times in an hour, to ask or confirm the days they had exercise. They typically lived alone and managed their own schedules; however, adding exercise sessions revealed their inability to manage a schedule. We tried multiple strategies such as calendars and reminder calls, which worked for some but not all. Ultimately, some participants dropped out of the study. In retrospect, we may have been able to engage them better if we had an open gym where they could come when they felt like it or provided exercise at their homes on a flexible schedule.

Physical Aggression

Physical aggression was extremely rare in our participants. One such event was reported to us by Gregory, the husband and caregiver of Caroline, a participant. Caroline and Gregory were at a friend's house; they had visited the friend many times and knew the neighborhood quite well. At one point during the day, Gregory realized that he had not seen Caroline for a little while and started to look for her in the house and on the street. He could not find her anywhere. He called her phone, but she did not answer. Even though they knew the neighborhood, he was still very worried about her.

Caroline returned to the house on her own about 45 minutes later. Gregory was beside himself with worry, questioned her about where she had gone, and told her not to leave without telling him where she was going. This made Caroline quite angry; she said she felt as though she was not being treated with the respect due to an adult. She balled up her fists and used harsh, threatening language. Gregory's attempts to calm her just enraged her further. She even knocked over a lamp and pushed a picture frame off the wall. Gregory decided that, for everyone's safety, he should call the police.

Gregory did a good job explaining to the police that his wife had cognitive impairment and was not armed. He just needed a respected, authoritative presence to help restore calm. He also suggested to the police that, when they talk with her, they should act as if they were "on her side" and say something like, "I think your husband may have overreacted a bit. Can you tell me what is going on?" The police spoke with her with respect, and she felt that they agreed that she was not in the wrong. The police calmed her and restored peace. Gregory also learned a lesson about the tone of voice to use with his wife and pass the lesson to us.

Socially Inappropriate Behavior

Leland lives at home with his wife. Leland had multiple careers, which he enjoyed talking about during exercise. He had a great sense of humor and loved to laugh and make witty puns. He loved his exercise sessions because they got him out of the house with someone new to talk to.

Around the fifth month of his participation in the study, I picked him up for exercise. When I rang the doorbell, he came to the door in just a bath towel. His wife called down the hallway that he would need to skip that day because he was nowhere near ready to go. In the next session, Leland told me that I should warn him the next time I came to his house. When I asked why, he said, "I could wear a smaller towel." I recognized this as socially inappropriate behavior and replied with, "Fully clothed is fine" in a joking tone of voice. Leland thought this was hilarious, and we laughed together. I knew that response would work for Leland because I knew his personality and his sense of humor very well. This response successfully diffused the situation and did not cause Leland to feel any shame for making a socially inappropriate comment. I was able to easily steer the conversation in a different direction afterward. These strategies worked in subsequent similar situations.

Delusion

Jerome lives with his son, daughter-in-law, and granddaughter. Throughout his life, he was politically informed and engaged. His participation in our study was during the 2016 presidential election. He liked to talk about Hillary Clinton and other political figures from his life during exercise. Although our ABC-MESSS Tool suggests avoiding contentious topics like politics, I was not always successful in changing the topic with Jerome.

One day, Jerome told me a story about meeting Hillary Clinton and becoming friends with her. The story was that he had met a relative of hers who invited him back to the home for dinner, where he met and became friends with Hillary. He talked at length about this meeting. After asking his family, I learned that Jerome had never met her.

One day on the drive to an exercise session, Jerome and another participant, Katherine, were arguing loudly about politics. Katherine supported Donald Trump. Our driver tried her best to calm and distract them, but she was driving on the interstate and could not keep track of the conversation behind her. By the time they arrived at the YMCA, Jerome and Katherine had forgotten about their argument.

We decided to keep Katherine and Jerome separated from that point on. In the car, one sat in the front and one in the back; at the YMCA, I had another participant sit between them. Katherine was hard of hearing, so having this separation was enough to allow Jerome to talk freely without inciting a debate. I did not confront Jerome about his delusion, because it made Jerome feel good and was not distressing to others. I asked him questions about their friendship, which he excitedly answered. Jerome had a perfect exercise attendance.

Agitation

Delores lives in an apartment with her daughter, Jenny. Delores saw our study flyer and called us. During the in-person interview, she became quite agitated or angry when she could not answer questions. Jenny told us privately that Delores is much better in the mornings than in the afternoons, so we scheduled her exercise sessions for mornings.

In the first few weeks of exercise, Delores seemed irritated and agitated by things such as putting on her heart rate monitor or being asked about her exercise exertion. Because she always agreed to come to exercise and had no issues with cycling, it seemed that interaction was the sole trigger for agitation, so I kept conversation to a minimum, which helped a lot. Delores often questioned why she was there and who signed her up for the study. I tried to turn it into a joke, saying, "Actually, *you* are the one who called me to sign up!" to which Delores would irritably reply, "I must have been out of my mind."

A couple of months later, Delores's attitude changed 180 degrees. She began to smile and was not agitated at all. She told funny jokes and stories and was very kind. When I shared my puzzlement with Jenny, I learned that all Delores' behaviors coincided with the arrival and departure of a difficult relative who had been staying with them. On her last day of exercise, she even gave me a hug!

Key Messages

- Approach AD S.A.F.E.ly™ HAPI Tool is used to getting to know your clients, which is foundational for addressing their unique AD symptoms during exercise.
- HAPI stands for <u>H</u>ave the right attitude; <u>A</u>sk the family caregiver, <u>P</u>ick out a routine that works for everyone; and <u>I</u>nitiate on day one.
- Common cognitive symptoms during exercise include repetitive questioning, memory impairment, and impaired judgment; functional symptoms include difficulty with cycle use, walking and balance issues, toileting, and hydration; and BPSD includes anxiety, aggression, socially inappropriate behavior, and delusion.
- You can apply the Approach AD S.A.F.E.ly™ ABC-MESSS Tool to respond to AD symptoms.

The Beginning Scenarios

Now let us take a look at the opening scenarios. Joan had extreme anxiety about not being ready for pickup. An 8 a.m. pickup to avoid traffic also caused anxiety overnight. I reduced her overnight anxiety by moving her pickup time to early afternoon, but then she had sundowning on the ride home from exercise. I eventually settled on a late morning routine and was able to reduce, but not completely relieve, her anxiety.

David and Alex had a combination of symptoms that led to physical aggression. Alex had a touch of socially inappropriate behavior by not being able to discern other's reactions to his jokes and the offensive nature of some of his jokes. David's family confirmed that David had been losing his inhibition as well. This combination caused physical aggression. I kept them in separate exercise sessions afterward.

Catherine continued to strive for independence, which I respected by supporting her decision to go to the back door on her own and asking her to wave through the window. However, Catherine did not recognize her keys as the tools that would open the door and needed help. Our driver asked for permission to help before assisting. Such incidences are common with people who have Alzheimer's dementia (e.g., not knowing how to use their gym membership card at check-in). Hence, knowing your clients helps.

Jacob had a delusion that someone was moving his belongings. He believed that, while he was at the study, someone had gone into his bedroom and moved them. The delusion was real to him, so I validated it. I tried to manage his delusion by working with his facility staff to give reassurances, have someone guard his room, or set up a security camera but were unsuccessful. Perhaps being able to exercise at home might have worked.

Chapter 11

How Can I Promote Exercise Engagement for People with Alzheimer's Dementia?

*W*illiam, 84, lived in an assisted living facility. Our exercise specialist, Sarah, had been talking with us about how to motivate William to exercise harder. Despite having exercised for more than a month, William pedaled at a low speed and resistance. When prompted to increase his speed, he would do nothing, but smile with a triumphant look in his eyes. If Sarah increased his resistance, he slowed even more. William sometimes stopped cycling and told Sarah, "I think I am done today." A few months after William exited our study, Sarah spoke to his facility staff member about another *matter. The staff member said, "By the way, William keeps asking why he is not going to the exercise program anymore. He said he loved it so much."*

———————●———————●———————

Jenny, 78, had a history of head injury, depression, diabetes, diarrhea, and digestive problems. One day before an exercise session, our exercise specialist, Kaitlin, received a call from Jenny's caregiver saying that Jenny had fallen and was in the hospital. We learned that Jenny had fallen twice over the weekend. The first time, her caregiver could not get her up and called 911. Paramedics got Jenny up and felt it was unnecessary to take her to the hospital. Jenny fell again the following night when getting up from the bed. The caregiver again could not get her up and called 911. The paramedics found Jenny disoriented and took her to the hospital.

———————●———————●———————

Mark, 79, had a history of shortness of breath, difficulty falling asleep, depression, knee and shoulder replacement, and possible seizures. One day, Mark finished cycling and walked over to sit in a chair. As Kaitlin turned to put down the exercise log, she heard a thump and saw that Mark had fallen to the floor. After establishing that he was not hurt, Kaitlin helped him get up and into the chair. Mark said he was trying to turn the chair for a better view of a tennis game on TV and lost his balance. His back bumped against the cycle, but his head did not hit it or the floor. Kaitlin evaluated Mark for any injuries and noted a scrape on his back. Mark insisted that he was fine and was just embarrassed that he fell.

The above scenarios were unexpected events during our studies. When events like these occur, exercise providers who have been trained in working with people with Alzheimer's dementia make all the difference in evaluating the situation, communicating with the participants and their family caregivers, and coordinating care to ensure timely assessment of our participants by their health care providers and their ongoing, safe exercise engagement.

This chapter specifically addresses you as the exercise provider who plans and supervises exercise sessions for people with Alzheimer's dementia. You might identify yourself as a personal trainer, an aerobics instructor, or a health care professional such as a physician, nurse, occupational, physical, or recreational therapist, or exercise physiologist. Family caregivers and friends may also assume the role of an exercise provider if they want to work with their loved ones in this capacity.

In this chapter, you will learn about our Approach AD S.A.F.E.ly™ working with family caregivers using our BEIC Tool and your clients' health care providers. You will use our RECUSS Tool to motivate your clients to exercise. Next, you will become familiar with adapting exercise for specific deficits and setting up exercise logistics appropriate for the different phases of Alzheimer's disease (AD) and stages of Alzheimer's dementia. Last, you will be introduced to the FIT-AD™ Certificate Program, which gives you the knowledge and skills to become a Memory Loss Exercise Specialist.

How Can I Work with Family Caregivers?

Engaging people with Alzheimer's dementia in aerobic exercise is a collaborative work. In addition to your clients, your most important partners in ensuring ongoing, safe exercise engagement are their family caregivers and health care providers. Our Approach AD S.A.F.E.ly™ BEIC Tool provides you with four strategies to work with family caregivers. BEIC, pronounced "bake," stands for Befriend, Empathize, Identify, and Communicate. Let us discuss each strategy in detail.

Befriend

Working with family caregivers is essential for building your relationships with your clients. The caregivers can give you insight into your clients' personality before and after AD, specific AD symptoms and strategies to address them, levels of awareness about AD, communication changes, preferred and effective ways of communication, and likes and dislikes so you can build a relationship and friendship over time with your clients. You will likely find that you become friends with the caregivers as well. Through our studies, many caregivers have kept in contact with us after their participation in the study ended. We often see them at AD-related events, and it is like a reunion of old friends.

Empathize

You will find that you are in a unique position as the exercise provider. You have a deep understanding of your clients' symptoms, abilities, and limitations as well as the family caregivers' difficulties at home. Of importance, you are not a member of the family or their social circles. Because you are an "outsider," the caregivers may come to you with their frustrations as a caregiver. Many caregivers do not talk about their frustrations to their friends or families because they do not want to appear to speak poorly of or complain about a loved one with a disease. However, as someone outside the family and friend social groups, the caregivers may not have the same hesitation venting their frustrations to you.

It is important to take the time to be compassionate, listen, and empathize. Caregiving has joys and rewards, but also difficulties and frustrations. It is important for family caregivers to be able to talk about them with someone they trust, although you may not provide any "real" help to solve their problems. This is not to say that family caregivers no longer love your clients, only that caregiving can be difficult and emotionally exhausting and take a toll. Being able to talk about it and getting some respite time (e.g., during the exercise session) is very important for the well-being of family caregivers.

Identify

Identify the point of contact for different issues you may face in working with your clients. If your clients live at home with family, the family members likely will be your first point of contact. Some clients may have a volunteer, hired help, or friend who visits them regularly. It is prudent to know these people's names, phone numbers, and the days of visits with your clients. If your clients live in a facility such as an independent apartment building or a memory care facility, it is important to have the names and phone numbers of the front desks, nursing stations, or facility managers who have daily contact with your clients.

For example, suppose your client, LaVonne, lives alone in an assisted living facility. A facility staff member, Maggie, helps her with some activities of daily living, and an adult son, Gordon, is the family caregiver and visits once a week. Gordon initially talked to LaVonne to have her start an exercise program. You arranged the initial exercise schedule with Gordon, but then Gordon wanted you to work with Maggie because she knows more about LaVonne and the facility's activity schedule and can help keep LaVonne on time for exercise.

Communicate

Effective communication is essential for exercise sessions to run smoothly. This includes communication about exercise days and times, transportation, cancellations, delays, and other things that may pop up during the course of the exercise sessions. It is important to know family caregivers' preferred mode of communication so you know that your communication will get through. The caregivers also need to know your preferred mode of communication. For example, our exercise specialists prefer that family caregivers call their cell phones rather than office phones, especially on days of an exercise session, to ensure timely communication.

In addition, we have found it useful to always use two modes of communication when discussing schedules. Often, we call family caregivers to set up exercise schedules and then follow up with an email with the schedule we created so they can reference it later. For those who prefer emails only, we often send a separate email once we have decided on the schedules so that it is easy for family caregivers to reference.

How Can I Work with Health care Providers?

The purpose of working with your clients' health care providers is to ensure exercise safety. The providers whom you will work with are cardiologists or primary care providers such as physicians and nurse practitioners but might also include nurses, social workers, and facility staff. Depending on your clients' preferences, you may interact with their health care providers directly. If you have permission from your clients or their surrogate decision-makers, you can contact the providers directly. If you do not have permission, you need to advise your clients and their family caregivers to follow up with the providers to get the information you need, such as medical clearance or consultation on a new symptom.

Obtain Medical Clearance

When medical clearance is required for your clients during pre-exercise health screening, you need to facilitate the process of getting it. If your clients are being treated for cardiovascular conditions, they likely have a cardiologist. In this case, medical clearance from the cardiologist is needed. If your clients have neither a cardiovascular condition nor a cardiologist, the primary care providers can give medical clearance.

Give the providers sufficient information to make medical clearance easy for everyone. You can prepare a medical clearance form or use our form. Our form contains two parts: Part 1 is a synopsis and Part 2 is a checklist completed by the providers. Part 1 should contain your client's name, date of birth, and phone number; planned exercise dose (frequency, intensity, and session duration); and reasons for requesting medical clearance. Part 2 asks about any contraindications, concerns, and specific recommendations for exercise. Part 2 could include a checklist of options such as 1) Can exercise at the target dose, 2) Can exercise in supervised rehabilitation settings only, and 3) No exercise. You could ask your clients to bring the medical clearance form to an appointment for the providers to complete. If you have your clients' permission and a fax machine, you can fax the form, along with the written permission, and ask the providers to fax back the completed form.

Address Changing Medical Conditions

If your clients report or you notice any changes in their medical conditions, such as unusual high blood pressure and new or worsening symptoms, keep everyone informed. However, always get your clients' permission before you communicate with family caregivers or health care providers. Ask your clients with whom they prefer you to communicate. To avoid prying into personal affairs, keep your communications professional and always focus on your clients' safety.

Let us continue to use LaVonne as the example. After obtaining LaVonne's permission, you communicated with Gordon and her nurse: "In the past few days, LaVonne's blood pressure has been a bit higher than her normal blood pressure. Have there been any changes that may be causing this?" It turned out that LaVonne's provider recently adjusted her medication.

How Can I Motivate People to Exercise?

Despite the well-established exercise benefits, a sedentary lifestyle is common, and motivating your clients to begin ongoing exercise engagement is critical. In our studies, we have found that what motivates one participant may not motivate another. Some of our participants were self-motivated to attend the exercise sessions. They got ready for their exercise sessions with little or no help from their family caregivers and needed only reminders of when to get ready. Others needed an external influence to motivate them to go, but once they arrived at the exercise facility, they usually enjoyed the exercise. A small number of participants did not like exercise and quit after a few sessions. You can use our Approach AD S.A.F.E.ly™ RECUSS Tool to motivate your clients. RECUSS, which is pronounced "recess," stands for Rely on rapport with your client, Establish an enjoyable environment, Capitalize on social support, Understand your influence, Sing praises for effort, and Support family caregivers.

Rely on Rapport with Your Client

We have found that many research participants were motivated to be ready on time because they did not want to appear rude or keep us waiting. Many family caregivers have relayed that they used us as a major motivator, such as "The university car will be here in 15 minutes! Can you put your shoes and coat on?" If your clients think of you as their friend who they get to hang out with for an hour, it will help them stick to the exercise schedules. Before and after an exercise session, socialize with your clients while getting them ready for the session or go home to foster your rapport. This may also give you additional insights into motivation strategies for your clients.

Establish an Enjoyable Environment

Establishing an enjoyable environment goes all the way back to your initial encounter with your clients. It depends on how well you did your assessment about getting to know them. To make exercise enjoyable, talk about things your clients are interested in at their communication and cognition levels and understand their personalities. This is especially important when creating small-group exercise sessions.

A recent study found that motivation *during* exercise was higher than motivation *to attend* a session in people with dementia, which could be caused by a number of factors. The exercise program was individualized to each participant. The exercise schedules were consistent, with the same participants in a group. The exercise providers established a routine and familiarization. Our Approach AD S.A.F.E.ly™ protocol includes all these strategies.

If your clients never had much interest in exercise during their life, you may need to focus extra efforts on creating a fun atmosphere during exercise. On the other extreme, if your clients were avid exercisers, they may be motivated already; however, it is still important to cultivate a fun atmosphere and relationship with them to help prevent the loss of interest, which may occur as AD progresses.

Capitalize on Social Support

Solicit help and encouragement from your clients' family members, friends, and social network. If they are committed to getting your clients to exercise, your clients will likely stick to it. Some of our participants' families tied fun events to exercise milestones, such as joining friends for lunch or dinner after an exercise session. Other families show their support by coming to the exercise sessions occasionally, especially when friends visit from out of town.

Understand Your Influence

As described in Chapter 9, depression and apathy are common in people with Alzheimer's dementia. It can be easy for them to "blow-off" a family member who tries to engage them in an activity; however, it is much harder for them to blow off an outsider, especially if you have taken the time to arrange the exercise sessions for them.

Sing Praises for Effort

Celebrating and praising your clients' efforts during the exercise sessions can motivate them to keep working hard and return to the next session. These efforts are often easy to identify. For example, your client exercised five minutes longer than two days ago; reached a higher intensity level, as evidenced by heart rates or perceived exertion; or arrived at the exercise session on time. Praise for the efforts, which is advocated by the Positive Coaching Alliance, is increasingly recognized as an important motivation strategy for exercise and sports.

Support Family Caregivers

Even when caregivers know that the exercise sessions are fun and their loved ones enjoy exercise, it can be very frustrating for them to get someone out the door who argue with them. Some participants loved to exercise and were always excited and happy once they left home; yet when their caregivers tried to help them get ready, they resisted, yelled, and even refused to go, which was very hard on the caregivers. If the caregivers are having a difficult time, you may suggest arranging for someone outside the family (e.g., a friend or a volunteer from church) to be an exercise partner.

What Are Other AD-Related Changes?

As AD progresses, you may notice other changes in your clients that may affect exercise participation, including changes in motor skills, perception, and social cognition, as well as sundowning. You need to watch for these changes and adapt exercise to maximize its effectiveness and safety.

Motor and Perception Changes

AD affects the motor nervous system, which leads to deficits in muscle control, decreased senses of movement and body perception, and reduced lean muscle mass. These changes can cause unsteady gait and balance problems, placing people with Alzheimer's dementia at an increased risk for falls. As a result, certain exercise types, such as treadmill walking, can be dangerous. Seated and stationary aerobic exercises such as cycle ergometry are safe and smart choices.

In Chapter 2, you learned that AD most notably destroys the cholinergic neurons and their neurotransmitter, acetylcholine. Not only are cholinergic neurons important in brain function, but they are also found throughout the human body. The cholinergic neurons are important regulators of the cardiovascular system, including heart rate control. Disruption in normal cholinergic neuron function is commonly called autonomic dysfunction. A common sign of autonomic dysfunction is an insufficient heart rate response to exercise in the absence of heart rate-altering medications. If you notice that your client's heart rates do not increase with increasing exercise intensity and your client is not on a heart rate-altering medication, it may indicate autonomic dysfunction, a medical condition that requires medical clearance.

If autonomic dysfunction is present, exercise intensity must be based on a subjective method rather than heart rate. Furthermore, autonomic dysfunction may predispose your client to dizziness while standing up, fainting, and falls. Hence, it is important to assess blood pressure during and after exercise; extend the cool-down to help prevent post-exercise low blood pressure, and encourage slow standing from seated exercise.

Social Cognition Changes

AD affects brain areas controlling social cognition. As discussed in Chapter 9, a change in social cognition can show up as disinhibition, such as behaviors outside of the acceptable social norm, insensitivity to social standards, and decision-making without regard to safety. Social cognition can decline gradually or suddenly as AD progresses, which can influence exercise engagement.

As an exercise provider, you are responsible for creating a safe exercise environment for your clients. When you organize a small-group exercise session, consider compatibility among your clients based on factors such as personality and anticipate changes over time. For instance, say two of your clients initially enjoyed exercising together. Over time, one of them experiences a decline in social cognition and begins to make comments that the other client finds offensive. When this happens, consider regrouping or offering one-on-one sessions.

Sundowning

Because routine is very important to people with Alzheimer's dementia, try to schedule exercise sessions at the same time of the day and adapt schedules as needed. Some people with Alzheimer's dementia experience sundowning, which means that their AD symptoms worsen in the late afternoon and early evening. Exercise in the morning or early afternoon works better for these people. This is also the time of the day when humans are most alert due to the circadian rhythm.

What Logistics Do I Need to Consider?

In previous chapters, you have learned the different person-centered strategies in starting, progressing, and engaging people with Alzheimer's dementia in an individualized aerobic exercise program. This section introduces more strategies specific to the different phases of AD and stages of Alzheimer's dementia before, during, and after an exercise session. Table 11.1 provide an overview of the general strategies that will work for all phases of AD and stages of Alzheimer's dementia.

Table 11.1. General Strategies Across AD Phases

Occasion	Engagement Strategies
Before exercise	Set up exercise sessions workable for a client's routine
	Arrange transportation to the exercise facility
	Stuff a gym bag (emergency contact, exercise logbook, a change of clothes, towel, water bottle, snacks, if have diabetes, also blood sugar testing kit, and orange juice or glucose tablet)
	Make reminder communications (exercise time/location, meal 30 minutes before, exercise clothe and shoes, and changes in conditions)
During exercise	Meet at the bus stop, entrance, or check-in desk
	Answer repetitive questions as new questions
	Suggest bathroom use before and after exercise
	Demonstrate what you want the client to do
	Remind the client to sip water every 5-10 minutes
	Encourage and praise for efforts and progress
	Monitor unmet needs, signs, and symptoms
After exercise	Update logbook (exercise summary and plan for the next session)
	Communicate and coordinate care if needed
	Provide regular updates to the family caregiver about exercise progress and responses or any strategies that may help the caregiver
	Celebrate exercise milestones regularly to keep the client motivated
	Provide exercise summary for upcoming medical appointment

Preclinical AD & Mild Cognitive Impairment

This section addresses you as the person with preclinical AD or mild cognitive impairment due to AD. You are independent in your daily activities and can exercise on your own without an exercise provider. However, we do recommend that you establish a relationship with an exercise provider for two main reasons. First, the exercise provider can assess your fitness, establish your exercise program, and adjust your exercise program as your condition changes. You can choose the frequency of interactions with your exercise provider such as quarterly, semi-annually, or annually as you see fit. Second, if you experience cognitive decline and progress to Alzheimer's dementia over time, you will eventually need an exercise provider to supervise your exercise. It is beneficial to have someone who already knows you and with whom you like to work.

Before an exercise session

If you start on your own, make sure to complete the Approach AD S.A.F.E.ly™ pre-exercise health screening and set up your exercise goals for each session as outlined in Chapter 7. Exercising on your own gives you the maximum flexibility in your exercise schedule and location (e.g., at home, in the park, inside a mall, or at a gym). However, it does not mean you have to exercise alone unless you want to. Enlisting your families and friends to exercise together may keep you motivated and engaged in the long run.

Before you head to an exercise session, wear snug-fitting exercise shoes with good grips and exercise outfits (exercise pants or shorts and shirt). In your gym bag, include a heart rate monitor if you use one, a copy of the rating of perceived exertion scale, an exercise logbook and pen (for recording exercise achievements), a change of clothes for after-exercise, a towel for wiping up sweat during exercise and after taking a shower, a water bottle for hydration, some snacks after exercise in case your blood sugar level drops, your gym pass if evidence of membership is required, and the emergency phone numbers for family and health care providers. If you have diabetes, make sure to include the blood sugar testing kit and a bottle of orange juice or something similar that can increase your blood sugar level quickly if you experience low blood sugar.

During an exercise session

If this is your first exercise session, take your time to get familiar with the physical environment, such as the location of the locker room, bathroom, water fountain, and emergency exit. Use the bathroom if needed, fill your water bottle, and get everything you need set up. For example, put on your heart rate monitor, place your rating of perceived exertion scale on the console of the exercise equipment, get your exercise music or book ready, and keep your exercise logbook and pen handy for recording. Follow your exercise goal for the session to warm up.

During exercise, closely monitor your physical responses to exercise, such as your heart rate, perceived exertion, breathing, and ability to talk to stay within your target heart rate zone or rating of perceived exertion levels. Watch for any signs and symptoms of overexertion (review Chapter 8 as needed). It is perfectly fine to adjust your session goal down if you are having a bad day, but never push for a higher goal than planned during a session, even if you feel you can do it. Sip water every five to 10 minutes to keep hydrated, whether or not you are thirsty.

You can exercise continuously until you reach your planned session duration at moderate intensity or exercise in several short intervals. For example, instead of doing 50 minutes of continuous cycling, you can cycle for 10 to 15 minutes at a time with a break in between. Upon completing your planned duration of exercise at moderate intensity, make sure to cool down.

After an exercise session

The cool-down period can also be used for recording exercise achievements, such as exercise duration, intensity, and distance, in the exercise logbook. A quick note such as "5/20/2019: cycled for 35 minutes at resistance three and 50 revolutions per minute for six miles" is sufficient. If you want to go further, write down your peak heart rate, peak perceived exertion level, signs and symptoms during exercise, and any reminders about what to do for the next exercise session.

The exercise logbook is also a great way to celebrate your exercise achievements. Our research participants took great pride in their achievements and shared their exercise logbooks with family and friends. We also give a Certificate of Completion to participants once they finish the six-month exercise program as a souvenir, so find a way to celebrate your milestones.

Take time to unwind by using the bathroom, drinking water, changing into the dry clothes in your gym bag, eating a snack before leaving the facility, or socializing with other exercisers or facility staff. Listen to your body, and observe any reactions to exercise afterward.

Mild-to-Moderate Alzheimer's Dementia

We strongly recommend supervised aerobic exercise for people with Alzheimer's dementia due to AD's impact on judgment and decision-making. Logistically, people with Alzheimer's dementia may not be able to coordinate exercise schedules and/or drive to and from exercise facilities. The strategies described for people with preclinical AD and mild cognitive impairment still apply to people with Alzheimer's dementia, but they need to be facilitated or carried out by the exercise providers. Hence, this section is addressed to the exercise providers. In the opening scenarios at the beginning of this chapter, you saw that we called the exercise providers in our studies "exercise specialists" because they have been educated to work with people with Alzheimer's dementia.

Before an exercise session

In our studies with older adults with mild-to-moderate Alzheimer's dementia, our exercise specialists coordinate exercise schedules and transportation with the participants and their family caregivers. We provide transportation for all study-related activities. In real life, you need to think creatively with your clients about transportation, unless you do home visits. Potential options include public transit, if convenient and easy; mobility services provided by nonprofit organizations or a state's health department; transportation provided by family caregivers or friends; shared rides; or taxis.

Get to know your clients, create a communication plan, and communicate in a way that is sensitive to the clients' communication deficits (review Chapter 6 about stage-specific communication changes in Alzheimer's dementia). It is particularly important to ask your clients how they prefer to communicate when they have trouble finding words. Do they prefer that you tell them the words or that you wait to let them come up with them? Should phone calls, texts, or emails be the primary means for reminders of the date, time, and location of an exercise session, meals at least 30 minutes before the session, and any changes in the exercise schedules or your clients' conditions? We recommend that you always carry your clients' emergency contact information for their family and primary care providers. Keep a stock of glucose tablets, which can be purchased over the counter at a pharmacy, if your clients have diabetes.

Help orient your clients. Before your clients know you, tape a photo of you to the exercise logbooks. Inadequate dietary intake may present a challenge because your clients may have increasing difficulty using utensils and may need help to eat. Be cognizant of the risk for falls because gait changes become increasingly common as well.

Unless one-on-one exercise sessions are specifically requested, it is always a good idea to create small-group exercise sessions to engage two or three clients together. Our participants have formed new friendships and were motivated to see their friends and exercise together.

During an exercise session

No matter how your clients arrive, meet them at the door, parking lot, bus stop, or check-in desk and orient them to who you are, where they are, and what you will do together. As a conversation starter, do a quick assessment to see if your clients have done any exercise, their responses to the last exercise session, any new signs or symptoms, and health condition or medication changes since you last saw them.

As you walk with your clients to the exercise room or equipment, observe their gait and posture to assess their fall risk. Our exercise specialists were taught to walk a bit sideways next to our participants, which allows them to observe participants' gait. If a client is at risk for falls, the exercise specialist worked with the family to identify fall-prevention strategies and used a gait belt, if necessary.

Once your clients arrive at the exercise equipment, explain and demonstrate how to use the exercise equipment and the exercise you want them to do step by step. If needed, give physical assistance such as helping put their feet into the strap of the pedals on a recumbent stationary cycle.

If you supervise several clients exercising in a group, get everyone ready first by having all your clients sit on their recumbent stationary cycles. You can space out the start time for cycling by having one client start to pedal for a minute or two before having the next client start (review Chapter 10 for a detailed spacing illustration). Such spacing will give you enough time to adjust exercise intensity and speed for each client without feeling hurried.

Tune into your clients' favorite TV shows or music to help them engage in exercise if they prefer. Monitor their responses to exercise, and record their exercise intensity and responses regularly, such as every 10 to 15 minutes, which will allow you to compare each client's progress and responses over time. Acknowledge exercise efforts and progress frequently and be on alert for unmet needs to address them right away.

After an exercise session

In addition to documenting exercise achievements, the exercise logbook is a great way for you to communicate with your clients and their family caregivers. Our exercise specialists write the date, time, and transportation arrangement for the next exercise session in the exercise log. If the next session has not yet been determined or they have noticed anything unusual or helpful, they write in the exercise logbook that they will contact the family caregivers to set up the next session or discuss their observations. Make sure to show your clients what you have written, and always follow up with an email, text, or phone call to the family caregivers in case they did not see what was written in the exercise logbook.

Establishing rapport and relationship with your clients is critical to their ongoing exercise engagement. Build in time for social interactions after the session. For example, wait with your clients for their rides home, share experiences, and learn about their eating habits, which will help you know your clients better and understand their nutritional status better. Many of our participants expressed that their friendship with our exercise specialists is one of the main reasons that they kept showing up for exercise sessions.

Severe Alzheimer's Dementia

People with severe Alzheimer's dementia may participate in aerobic exercise if they are mobile (not bed-bound). Strategies previously described for people with mild-to-moderate Alzheimer's dementia still apply but need to be modified for those with severe Alzheimer's dementia.

Before an exercise session

People with severe Alzheimer's dementia may be ambulatory or non-ambulatory. You need to assess their physical ability to select an appropriate exercise, such as arm cycle-ergometer exercise for clients who are not ambulatory. Interval exercise may be more appropriate than continuous exercise, especially for those with bowel and bladder issues or who are physically deconditioned. Breaks between exercise intervals can be used for hydration or a trip to the bathroom. You could also mix aerobic exercise with other exercises, such as range-of-motion activities.

During an exercise session

Pay close attention to nonverbal communications to gauge how much your clients enjoy the exercise. Seated exercises may help prevent falls, but be aware that people can still fall. Behavioral and psychological symptoms may appear but do not necessarily compromise exercise participation. We once had a participant who had visual hallucination (seeing another person who was not there). During exercise, he talked to that person frequently, which actually kept him going on the cycle.

Rely on nonverbal cues, signs, and symptoms for assessing exercise responses because people with severe Alzheimer's dementia have increasing difficulty with verbal communications. One of our participants with severe Alzheimer's dementia rarely spoke words. In the first month, when we asked whether she liked the exercise program, she did not give a verbal response. However, we began to notice a change in her facial expression over time. She began to respond to this question with a small smile.

After an exercise session

At this stage of Alzheimer's dementia, AD brain changes are severe and widespread, affecting many bodily functions. The goal of exercise engagement is to have your clients be as physically active as they can. Any exercise that your clients can participate in is better than none. Thus, after each exercise session, reflect on how well your clients were engaged in the session and adjust it accordingly for the next session.

Why Is It Important to Become a Specialist?

One of the hardest things we have to do is to inform our research participants that they have completed our exercise program. The participants and their family caregivers have consistently expressed their gratitude towards our staff, who really understand what they have been going through and how disappointed they are at not being able to continue. It is a true dilemma because family caregivers have noted tangible exercise benefits in their loved ones. However, there are few community-based options to keep the participants going after exiting our studies. The reasons for this dilemma are complex and multitude. One bottleneck that we chose to tackle was the lack of exercise providers who are educated to supervise people with Alzheimer's dementia in aerobic exercise.

Lack of Exercise Providers Trained in AD

We have previously distinguished between an exercise provider and an exercise specialist. An exercise provider is anyone who plans and supervises exercise sessions for other people. In contrast, we reserved the term "exercise specialists" for exercise providers trained in engaging people with Alzheimer's dementia in exercise, such as the exercise providers in our studies.

In the United States, the number of positions for fitness trainers and aerobics instructors alone is projected to grow at a faster than average pace. According to the U.S. Bureau of Labor Statistics, there were 299,200 positions for fitness trainers and aerobics instructors in 2016, and that number will increase to 329,200 by 2026. Training to become an exercise provider may include content on Alzheimer's dementia, but there is a lack of evidence-based programs on how to effectively and safely engage people with Alzheimer's dementia in aerobic exercise.

Traditionally, exercise providers have worked in the community (e.g., community centers, gyms, wellness centers, and rehabilitation centers). They are increasingly hired by senior facilities such as adult day centers and assisted living, memory care, and skilled nursing facilities. The anticipated growth of these facilities from 2015 to 2020 was estimated at 2.5% to 7%.

Most senior facilities offer some exercise programs that may or may not meet the weekly doses of exercise recommended for older adults. New high-end senior facilities often have a dedicated exercise room with state-of-the-art exercise equipment, but the equipment may not be used by people with Alzheimer's dementia due to reasons such as the lack of awareness of the importance of exercise for this population, staffing shortages, and concerns about exercise safety.

Need for Supervised Exercise

Mild Alzheimer's dementia is a critical stage for enacting advanced care planning such as financial and health power of attorney, advance directives, and ongoing exercise engagement. There is no doubt that some people with mild Alzheimer's dementia are fully capable of doing aerobic exercise on their own if exercise has been part of their lifestyle. However, even for them, supervised exercise is eventually needed as AD progresses over time.

The Alzheimer's Rx: Aerobic Exercise

For most people with Alzheimer's dementia, supervised exercise is essential to ensure safety and enjoyment. Cognitive impairment makes it difficult for them to remember or learn what to do, navigate the physical and social environments, monitor their exercise responses, or use the exercise equipment. As previously described in Chapter 6, they have different levels of awareness about their AD and its impact, which limits their insight about their abilities and limitations. In the exercise sessions, we have observed the disconnect between the subjective ratings of perceived exertion and objective measures of exercise responses in our research participants. It is less a concern when a participant overrated exertion level when the objective measures indicated less intense exercise. The other disconnect, a low rating of exertion but signs and symptoms of overexertion, such as profuse sweating, severe shortness of breath, and an inability to speak a sentence without catching their breath several times, put our exercise specialists on high alert. They helped the participants slow down, reduce the resistance level, or both.

In the past, there was a misconception that people with Alzheimer's dementia have a brain condition but are otherwise healthy. This has turned out to be far from the truth. Multimorbidity (the presence of two or more chronic conditions) often affects people with Alzheimer's dementia. On average, people with dementia have 2.5 chronic conditions, are on five or more drugs, and are three times more likely than their peers with intact cognition to be hospitalized due to these conditions. Almost all research participants in our studies have had a unique combination of medical conditions. No two participants have been similar, even if they were the same age, sex, and educational level. Each participant also had his or her own unique clusters of cognitive, functional, behavioral, and psychological symptoms as well as family and social contexts, which change over time. The medical conditions and AD symptoms together present distinct barriers to exercise engagement for each participant.

Benefits of Being Educated about AD

Supervising people with Alzheimer's dementia in exercise is not a job for exercise providers who are not properly trained. Working with this population in exercise requires special skills and is extremely rewarding, but can be emotionally taxing, as testified by our exercise specialists like Kaitlin Kelly, a co-author of this book. At some exercise sessions, Kaitlin answered the same question 10 to 20 times. Behavioral and psychological symptoms could be very challenging to address as well. A few research participants were outright hostile to Kaitlin and told her point-blank, "I do not like you." One participant had social disinhibition and used offensive language to describe women in conversations with Kaitlin. Some participants had trouble with bladder control and had to go to the bathroom every 10 to 15 minutes, while Kaitlin had to watch the participants still exercising *and* the participant who had gone to the bathroom. Despite the challenges, Kaitlin eventually won over these participants. Almost all of the participants appreciated Kaitlin's company. Many called her a friend or adopted family member. Kaitlin has repeatedly told her family and friends that she has the best job ever.

Family caregivers have often told us that we have the best staff. There is no doubt that our staff members are great people. Their greatness has been enhanced by their training and support in understanding AD and exercise as well as working with people with Alzheimer's dementia, their family caregivers, and health care providers.

How Do I Become a Specialist?

Motivated by our research participants and family caregivers who demanded ongoing exercise participation, we took the first step in making exercise available to people with Alzheimer's dementia in 2016 by developing the FIT-AD™ Certificate Program. The FIT-AD™ Certificate Program filled the void in evidence-based educational programs to help exercise providers understand what AD is, how it affects people, and how to engage people affected by AD safely in aerobic exercise on an ongoing basis.

The FIT-AD™ Certificate Program

The FIT-AD™ Certificate Program is one of a kind because it is based on our years of aerobic exercise research in people with Alzheimer's dementia since 2005. It was approved by the American College of Sports Medicine for continuing education credits for exercise providers. The FIT-AD™ Certificate Program uses active learning and unfolding case studies to provide the knowledge, skills, and tools for exercise providers to understand AD and apply our Approach AD S.A.F.E.ly™ protocol to get to know people affected by AD, communicate with them effectively, conduct pre-exercise health screening, design individualized aerobic exercise programs, set up exercise sessions, engage them in ongoing exercise, address changes in AD symptoms and medical conditions, and work with family caregivers and health care providers. Exercise providers who complete the program earn a certificate of completion as a Memory Loss Exercise Specialist at the basic or advanced level.

Process for Obtaining the Certificate

To become a Memory Loss Exercise Specialist at the basic level, you need to complete Part I of the FIT-AD™ Certificate Program and obtain a score of at least 80% on the certificate test. Part I is an online program composed of four modules, including 1) Understand AD; 2) Start People Affected by AD in Exercise; 3) Progress Exercise to the Target Level; and 4) Maintain Exercise as AD Worsens. Each module involves interactive presentations, resources, and self-study quizzes. It takes about eight to 12 hours of study to master the content.

To receive the certificate at the advanced level, you need to participate in Part II, a 7.5-hour in-person workshop to gain advanced skills to work with people affected by AD. You will learn and practice key skills from Part I through case studies. We are currently seeking funding to revise the Part I modules and make Part II available online to ultimately make the FIT-AD™ Certificate Program nationally and internationally available to increase the cadre of exercise specialists who can help make aerobic exercise widely accessible and a standard treatment for people with Alzheimer's dementia.

Key Messages

- People with preclinical AD or mild cognitive impairment can follow our Approach AD S.A.F.E.ly™ protocol to screen their conditions, design their exercise programs, and participate in aerobic exercise on their own.
- Supervised exercise is critical for people with Alzheimer's dementia due to the complexity of AD symptoms, altered awareness and judgment, and co-existing medical conditions.
- Exercise delivery needs to be adjusted if changes in motor skills, perception, social cognition, and sundowning are observed.
- Strategies before, during, and after an exercise session apply to all phases of AD and stages of Alzheimer's dementia but need to be modified and simplified over time based on each person's ability.

- The FIT-AD™ Certificate Program was designed to educate exercise providers to become Memory Loss Exercise Specialists at the basic or advanced level to increase exercise access for people affected by AD.

The Beginning Scenarios

Now, let us review the scenarios introduced at the beginning of this chapter. Were you surprised by the message relayed by William's facility staff member? We were all delightfully surprised that William remembered our program months later and even recalled that he enjoyed it. We tried every strategy in our toolbox, but truly nothing worked for more than a few sessions. He basically cycled at his will without making much progress in his exercise dose over six months. We knew he liked the program because he always agreed to come to the exercise sessions and had fun giving us "trouble" by not following our instructions.

Jenny's story illustrates the importance of working with family caregivers and health care providers to ensure timely communication, medical evaluation, and ongoing exercise participation and safety. Jenny's caregiver believed that both falls were due to poor balance, which her primary care provider confirmed. Jenny was medically cleared to resume exercise with us.

When Mark fell after cycling, Kaitlin alerted his caregiver right away about the fall and the need to watch for signs of infection. Kaitlin evaluated Mark again before he left and instructed other staff about Mark's fall risk and prevention strategies. In subsequent sessions, Kaitlin continued to monitor his scrape until it healed.

We hope Jenny's and Mark's fall incidents give you at least a shallow glimpse of the daily challenges that people with Alzheimer's dementia and their family caregivers face and put you on high alert for the prevalence of falls in this population. In fact, more than 60%

of older adults with Alzheimer's dementia fall every year, a rate three times higher than in those without Alzheimer's dementia. Falls lead to many poor health outcomes, such as increased death, nursing home placement, and health care costs. Many personal and environmental factors contribute to falls, with postural and gait instability the main reasons. AD brain changes interrupt the awareness of movement and sensory inputs that regulate equilibrium and gait. We put Jenny and Mark on fall alert and initiated fall prevention procedures.

Epilogue

Growing up, I was a sedentary and nerdy kid. I loved to study and worked through practice books one after another. My mom complained that I studied too much. I actually was pretty good at sports such as swimming, ice skating, and volleyball but did not do them often. I exercised from time to time but did not become a serious exerciser and firm believer until I started to research aerobic exercise.

My team and I strongly believe in aerobic exercise's potential for modifying the abnormal brain changes caused by Alzheimer's disease (AD) and AD's clinical course based on the converging research evidence from the various disciplines described in this book. This belief may have colored our interpretations of the research findings, although we strived to be as objective as possible.

Despite our passion for aerobic exercise and people affected by AD, we do not want to mislead you to think that aerobic exercise can prevent or cure AD by itself. However, we do think that aerobic exercise is essential for allowing other interventions to work optimally. Aerobic exercise, along with drugs and other lifestyle interventions that target diet, sleep, cardiovascular conditions and risk factors, cognitive training, and social engagement may generate greater effects than aerobic exercise alone. Experts have estimated that at least a third of all AD cases can be attributed to modifiable risk factors.

To this end, I thought about testing the effects of combining aerobic exercise with other interventions while running a study in 2010. My "plus one" pick was cognitive training, drugs, and diet, but life was busy, and time slid by. In fall 2015, I taught a research method course to our PhD students and shared my idea. A student, Joseph Alexander, was very intrigued and said, "You should meet my brilliant friend, Vankee Lin, at the University of Rochester. I think your work really complements each other." He was true to his word and emailed me Vankee's contact information. I contacted Vankee, and we met at the annual conference of the Gerontological Society of America that November. Long story short, our first two-site clinical trial, Efficacy and Mechanisms of Combined Aerobic Exercise and Cognitive Training (ACT) in MCI or the ACT Trial, was funded by the National Institute on Aging of the National Institutes of Health in September 2017. We began recruiting participants in June 2018.

Over the years, I have met researchers and clinicians who thought that the evidence for aerobic exercise in AD was not strong or conclusive enough for making a recommendation for treatment, but we disagree. On average, people with Alzheimer's dementia have lower aerobic fitness than peers without dementia, have 2.5 chronic conditions, and are taking five or more drugs, which can all be improved by aerobic exercise. Yes, the evidence is mixed, and the number of high-quality aerobic exercise trials are limited. Many unanswered questions merit further investigation: What is the optimal dose of aerobic exercise for AD prevention and treatment? Is there a limit to aerobic exercise's effects where more is not better? Who will most likely benefit from aerobic exercise? How does aerobic exercise affect AD brain changes in humans? However, does this mean that we should continue to tell people at risk for or affected AD, "Sorry, there is really nothing I can do for you?" Absolutely not. We believe that many evidence-based interventions can improve brain health, AD symptoms and experiences, functional independence, and quality of life.

Say that future findings overwhelmingly indicate that aerobic exercise has no cognitive benefits at all. So what? People who exercised would still reap all the other health benefits of aerobic exercise. Let us assume the worst-case scenario: We find that aerobic exercise hastens the progression of Alzheimer's dementia and that people with Alzheimer's dementia who exercise end up with a shorter life expectancy than those who do not. Will the tradeoff between exercise benefits and life expectancy be acceptable? We do not know about you, but for us, exercise means being able to be functionally independent for longer and have a better quality of life for a shorter number of years, which is worth way more than having a long and dependent life.

No matter which camp you are in (exercise, undecided, or no exercise), we hope you have found this book informative and interesting to read. It is our hope that you have a better appreciation of AD and how it affects people and families. The next time you meet someone who seems to have cognitive issues, perhaps you will be more willing to lend a hand and make our communities more dementia-friendly. For that, we thank you for reading this book!

— Fang Yu

References

Chapter 1

Albert, M. S., DeKosky, S. T., Dickson, D., Dubois, B., Feldman, H. H., Fox, N. C., . . . Phelps, C. H. (2011). The diagnosis of mild cognitive impairment due to Alzheimer's disease: Recommendations from the National Institute on Aging-Alzheimer's Association workgroups on diagnostic guidelines for Alzheimer's disease. *Alzheimer's & Dementia, 7*(3), 270-279.

Association, A. P. (2013). *Diagnostic and statistical manual of mental disorders* (5th ed.). Arlington, VA: American Psychiatric Assocation.

Craik, F. I., Salthouse, T. A. (2011). *The Handbook of Aging and Cognition* (3rd ed.). New York, NY: Psychology Press.

Drag, L. L., & Bieliauskas, L. A. (2010). Contemporary review 2009: cognitive aging. *Journal of Geriatric Psychiatry and Neurology, 23*(2), 75-93. doi:10.1177/0891988709358590

Driscoll, I., Davatzikos, C., An, Y., Wu, X., Shen, D., Kraut, M., & Resnick, S. M. (2009). Longitudinal pattern of regional brain volume change differentiates normal aging from MCI. *Neurology, 72*(22), 1906-1913. doi:10.1212/WNL.0b013e3181a82634

Dubois, B., Feldman, H. H., Jacova, C., Dekosky, S. T., Barberger-Gateau, P., Cummings, J., . . . Scheltens, P. (2007). Research criteria for the diagnosis of Alzheimer's disease: Revising the NINCDS-ADRDA criteria. *Lancet Neurology, 6*(8), 734-746. doi:10.1016/S1474-4422(07)70178-3

Dubois, B., Feldman, H. H., Jacova, C., Hampel, H., Molinuevo, J. L., Blennow, K., . . . Cummings, J. L. (2014). Advancing research diagnostic criteria for Alzheimer's disease: The IWG-2 criteria. *Lancet Neurology, 13*(6), 614-629. doi:10.1016/S1474-4422(14)70090-0

Fletcher, E., Gavett, B., Harvey, D., Farias, S. T., Olichney, J., Beckett, L., . . . Mungas, D. (2018). Brain volume change and cognitive trajectories in aging. *Neuropsychology, 32*(4), 436-449. doi:10.1037/neu0000447

Goldberg, T. E., Harvey, P. D., Wesnes, K. A., Snyder, P. J., & Schneider, L. S. (2015). Practice effects due to serial cognitive assessment: Implications for preclinical Alzheimer's disease randomized controlled trials. *Alzheimer's & Dementia (Amst), 1*(1), 103-111. doi:10.1016/j.dadm.2014.11.003

Harada, C. N., Natelson Love, M. C., & Triebel, K. L. (2013). Normal cognitive aging. *Clinics in Geriatric Medicine, 29*(4), 737-752. doi:10.1016/j.cger.2013.07.002

Jack, C. R., Albert, M. S., Knopman, D. S., McKhann, G. M., Sperling, R. A., Carrillo, M. C., . . . Phelps, C. H. (2011). Introduction to the recommendations from the National Institute on Aging-Alzheimer's Association workgroups on diagnostic guidelines for Alzheimer's disease. *Alzheimer's & Dementia, 7*(3), 257-262.

Jack, C. R., Jr., Bennett, D. A., Blennow, K., Carrillo, M. C., Dunn, B., Haeberlein, S. B., . . . Contributors. (2018). NIA-AA research framework: Toward a biological definition of Alzheimer's disease.

Alzheimer's & Dementia, 14(4), 535-562. doi:10.1016/j.jalz.2018.02.018

McKhann, G., Drachman, D., Folstein, M., Katzman, R., Price, D., & Stadlan, E. M. (1984). Clinical diagnosis of Alzheimer's disease: Report of the NINCDS-ADRDA Work Group under the auspices of Department of Health and Human Services Task Force on Alzheimer's Disease. *Neurology, 34*(7), 939-944.

McKhann, G. M., Knopman, D. S., Chertkow, H., Hyman, B. T., Jack, C. R., Jr., Kawas, C. H., . . . Phelps, C. H. (2011). The diagnosis of dementia due to Alzheimer's disease: Recommendations from the National Institute on Aging and the Alzheimer's Association workgroup. *Alzheimer's & Dementia, 7*(3), 263-269.

Peer, M., Salomon, R., Goldberg, I., Blanke, O., & Arzy, S. (2015). Brain system for mental orientation in space, time, and person. *Proceedings of the National Academy of Sciences of the United States of America, 112*(35), 11072-11077. doi:10.1073/pnas.1504242112

Petersen, R. C., Lundt, E. S., Therneau, T. M., Weigand, S. D., Knopman, D. S., Mielke, M. M., . . . Jack, C. R., Jr. (2019). Predicting progression to mild cognitive impairment. *Annals of Neurology, 85*(1), 155-160. doi:10.1002/ana.25388

Rabin, L. A., Smart, C. M., Crane, P. K., Amariglio, R. E., Berman, L. M., Boada, M., . . . Sikkes, S. A. (2015). Subjective cognitive decline in older adults: An overview of self-report measures used across 19 international research studies. *Journal of Alzheimer's Disease, 48 Suppl 1*, S63-86. doi:10.3233/JAD-150154

Salthouse, T. (2012). Consequences of age-related cognitive declines. *Annual Review of Psychology, 63*, 201-226. doi:10.1146/annurev-psych-120710-100328

Salthouse, T. A. (2010). Selective review of cognitive aging. *Journal of the International Neuropsychological Society, 16*(5), 754-760. doi:10.1017/S1355617710000706

Sperling, R. A., Aisen, P. S., Beckett, L. A., Bennett, D. A., Craft, S., Fagan, A. M., . . . Phelps, C. H. (2011). Toward defining the preclinical stages of Alzheimer's disease: Recommendations from the National Institute on Aging-Alzheimer's Association workgroups on diagnostic guidelines for Alzheimer's disease. *Alzheimer's & Dementia, 7*(3), 280-292.

Chapter 2

Ahmadian, N., Hejazi, S., Mahmoudi, J., & Talebi, M. (2018). Tau pathology of Alzheimer disease: Possible role of sleep deprivation. *Basic and Clinical Neuroscience, 9*(5), 307-316. doi:10.32598/bcn.9.5.307

Ayton, S., Wang, Y., Diouf, I., Schneider, J. A., Brockman, J., Morris, M. C., & Bush, A. I. (2019). Brain iron is associated with accelerated cognitive decline in people with Alzheimer pathology. *Molecular Psychiatry.* doi:10.1038/s41380-019-0375-7

Barnes, L. L., Capuano, A. W., Aiello, A. E., Turner, A. D., Yolken, R. H., Torrey, E. F., & Bennett, D. A. (2015). Cytomegalovirus infection and risk of Alzheimer disease in older black and white individuals. The *Journal of Infectious Diseases, 211*(2), 230-237. doi:10.1093/infdis/jiu437

Brickman, A. M., Tosto, G., Gutierrez, J., Andrews, H., Gu, Y., Narkhede, A., . . . Mayeux, R. (2018). An MRI measure of degenerative and cerebrovascular pathology in Alzheimer disease. *Neurology, 91*(15), e1402-e1412. doi:10.1212/WNL.0000000000006310

Cryan, J. F., & Dinan, T. G. (2012). Mind-altering microorganisms: The impact of the gut microbiota on brain and behaviour. *Nature Reviews of Neuroscience, 13*(10), 701-712. doi:10.1038/nrn3346

Reference

Dayon, L., Nunez Galindo, A., Wojcik, J., Cominetti, O., Corthesy, J., Oikonomidi, A., . . . Popp, J. (2018). Alzheimer disease pathology and the cerebrospinal fluid proteome. *Alzheimer's Research & Therapy, 10*(1), 66. doi:10.1186/s13195-018-0397-4

Finch, C. E., & Morgan, T. E. (2007). Systemic inflammation, infection, ApoE alleles, and Alzheimer disease: A position paper. *Current Alzheimer's Research, 4*(2), 185-189.

Fyfe, I. (2017). Alzheimer disease: Sex-specific inflammatory link to early Alzheimer pathology. *Nature Reviews Neurology, 13*(1), 5. doi:10.1038/nrneurol.2016.193

Gu, L., & Guo, Z. (2013). Alzheimer's Abeta42 and Abeta40 peptides form interlaced amyloid fibrils. *Journal of Neurochemistry, 126*(3), 305-311. doi:10.1111/jnc.12202

Huang, W. J., Zhang, X., & Chen, W. W. (2016). Role of oxidative stress in Alzheimer's disease. *Biomedical Reports, 4*(5), 519-522. doi:10.3892/br.2016.630

Hughes, T. M., Lockhart, S. N., & Smagula, S. F. (2018). Blood pressure's role in Alzheimer disease pathology. *The American Journal of Geriatric Psychiatry, 26*(1), 23-24. doi:10.1016/j.jagp.2017.09.019

Iqbal, K., Alonso Adel, C., Chen, S., Chohan, M. O., El-Akkad, E., Gong, C. X., . . . Grundke-Iqbal, I. (2005). Tau pathology in Alzheimer disease and other tauopathies. *Biochimica et Biophysica Acta, 1739*(2-3), 198-210. doi:10.1016/j.bbadis.2004.09.008

Jack, C. R., Albert, M. S., Knopman, D. S., McKhann, G. M., Sperling, R. A., Carrillo, M. C., . . . Phelps, C. H. (2011). Introduction to the recommendations from the National Institute on Aging-Alzheimer's Association workgroups on diagnostic guidelines for Alzheimer's disease. *Alzheimer's & Dementia, 7*(3), 257-262.

Jack, C. R., Jr., Barnes, J., Bernstein, M. A., Borowski, B. J., Brewer, J., Clegg, S., . . . Weiner, M. (2015). Magnetic resonance imaging in Alzheimer's Disease Neuroimaging Initiative 2. *Alzheimer's & Dementia, 11*(7), 740-756. doi:10.1016/j.jalz.2015.05.002 S1552-5260(15)00168-5 [pii]

Jack, C. R., Jr., Bennett, D. A., Blennow, K., Carrillo, M. C., Dunn, B., Haeberlein, S. B., . . . Contributors. (2018). NIA-AA Research Framework: Toward a biological definition of Alzheimer's disease. *Alzheimer's & Dementia, 14*(4), 535-562. doi:10.1016/j.jalz.2018.02.018

Kanatsu, K., & Tomita, T. (2017). Molecular mechanisms of the genetic risk factors in pathogenesis of Alzheimer disease. *Frontiers in Bioscience (Landmark Ed), 22*, 180-192.

Larsen, R. T., Christensen, J., Tang, L. H., Keller, C., Doherty, P., Zwisler, A. D., . . . Langberg, H. (2016). A systematic review and meta-Analysis comparing cardiopulmonary exercise test values obtained from the arm cycle and the leg cycle respectively in healthy adults. *International Journal of Sports Physical Therapy, 11*(7), 1006-1039.

Liu, Y., Braidy, N., Poljak, A., Chan, D. K. Y., & Sachdev, P. (2018). Cerebral small vessel disease and the risk of Alzheimer's disease: A systematic review. *Ageing Research Reviews, 47*, 41-48. doi:10.1016/j.arr.2018.06.002

Marrocco, I., Altieri, F., & Peluso, I. (2017). Measurement and clinical significance of biomarkers of oxidative stress in humans. *Oxidative Medicine and Cellular Longevity, 2017*, 6501046. doi:10.1155/2017/6501046

Mayer, F., Di Pucchio, A., Lacorte, E., Bacigalupo, I., Marzolini, F., Ferrante, G., . . . Vanacore, N. (2018). An estimate of attributable cases of Alzheimer disease and vascular dementia due to modifiable risk factors: The impact of primary prevention in

Europe and in Italy. *Dementia and Geriatric Cognitive Disorders Extra, 8*(1), 60-71. doi:10.1159/000487079

Moser, V. A., & Pike, C. J. (2017). Obesity accelerates Alzheimer-related pathology in APOE4 but not APOE3 Mice. *eNeuro, 4*(3). doi:10.1523/ENEURO.0077-17.2017

Neth, B. J., & Craft, S. (2017). Insulin resistance and Alzheimer's disease: Bioenergetic linkages. *Frontiers in Aging Neuroscience, 9*, 345. doi:10.3389/fnagi.2017.00345

Pruzin, J. J., Schneider, J. A., Capuano, A. W., Leurgans, S. E., Barnes, L. L., Ahima, R. S., . . . Arvanitakis, Z. (2017). Diabetes, hemoglobin A1C, and regional Alzheimer disease and infarct pathology. *Alzheimer Disease & Associated Disorders, 31*(1), 41-47. doi:10.1097/WAD.0000000000000172

Starling, S. (2018). Alzheimer disease: Blood-derived Abeta induces AD pathology. *Nature Reviews Neurology, 14*(1), 2. doi:10.1038/nrneurol.2017.164

Su, M., Naderi, K., Samson, N., Youssef, I., Fulop, L., Bozso, Z., . . . Davis, S. (2019). Mechanisms associated with type 2 diabetes as a risk factor for Alzheimer-related pathology. *Molecular Neurobiology*. doi:10.1007/s12035-019-1475-8

Talwar, P., Gupta, R., Kushwaha, S., Agarwal, R., Saso, L., Kukreti, S., & Kukreti, R. (2018). Viral induced oxidative and inflammatory response in Alzheimer's disease pathogenesis with identification of potential drug candidates: A systematic review using systems biology approach. *Current Neuropharmacology*. doi:10.2174/1570159X16666180419124508

Tatebe, H., Kasai, T., Ohmichi, T., Kishi, Y., Kakeya, T., Waragai, M., . . . Tokuda, T. (2017). Quantification of plasma phosphorylated tau to use as a biomarker for brain Alzheimer pathology: Pilot case-control studies including patients with

Alzheimer's disease and down syndrome. *Molecular Neurodegeneration, 12*(1), 63. doi:10.1186/s13024-017-0206-8

Varma, V. R., Oommen, A. M., Varma, S., Casanova, R., An, Y., Andrews, R. M., . . . Thambisetty, M. (2018). Brain and blood metabolite signatures of pathology and progression in Alzheimer disease: A targeted metabolomics study. *PLoS Medicine, 15*(1), e1002482. doi:10.1371/journal.pmed.1002482

Vergara, C., Houben, S., Suain, V., Yilmaz, Z., De Decker, R., Vanden Dries, V., . . . Brion, J. P. (2019). Amyloid-beta pathology enhances pathological fibrillary tau seeding induced by Alzheimer PHF in vivo. *Acta Neuropathology, 137*(3), 397-412. doi:10.1007/s00401-018-1953-5

Visser, P. J., & Tijms, B. (2017). Brain amyloid pathology and cognitive function: Alzheimer disease without dementia? *Journal of the Aermican Medical Association, 317*(22), 2285-2287. doi:10.1001/jama.2017.6895

Ziegler-Waldkirch, S., & Meyer-Luehmann, M. (2018). The role of glial cells and synapse loss in mouse models of Alzheimer's disease. *Frontiers in Cellular Neuroscience, 12*, 473. doi:10.3389/fncel.2018.00473

Chapter 3

Alzheimer's Association (2019). 2019 Alzheimer's disease facts and figures. Retrieved from https://www.alz.org/media/Documents/alzheimers-facts-and-figures-2019-r.pdf

Bediou, B., Ryff, I., Mercier, B., Milliery, M., Henaff, M. A., D'Amato, T., . . . Krolak-Salmon, P. (2009). Impaired social cognition in mild Alzheimer disease. *Journal of Geriatric Psychiatry and Neurology, 22*(2), 130-140. doi:10.1177/0891988709332939

Reference

Beeri, M. S., & Sonnen, J. (2016). Brain BDNF expression as a biomarker for cognitive reserve against Alzheimer disease progression. *Neurology,* *86*(8), 702-703. doi:10.1212/WNL.0000000000002389

Besser, L. M., Alosco, M. L., Ramirez Gomez, L., Zhou, X. H., McKee, A. C., Stern, R. A., . . . Kukull, W. A. (2016). Late-life vascular risk factors and Alzheimer disease neuropathology in individuals with normal cognition. *Journal of Neuropathology & Experimental Neurology,* *75*(10), 955-962. doi:10.1093/jnen/nlw072

Beydoun, M. A., Beydoun, H. A., Gamaldo, A. A., Teel, A., Zonderman, A. B., & Wang, Y. (2014). Epidemiologic studies of modifiable factors associated with cognition and dementia: Systematic review and meta-analysis. *BMC Public Health, 14*, 643. doi:10.1186/1471-2458-14-643

Blumenthal, J. A., Smith, P. J., Mabe, S., Hinderliter, A., Lin, P. H., Liao, L., . . . Sherwood, A. (2019). Lifestyle and neurocognition in older adults with cognitive impairments: A randomized trial. *Neurology,* *92*(3), e212-e223. doi:10.1212/WNL.0000000000006784

Borenstein, A. R., Copenhaver, C. I., & Mortimer, J. A. (2006). Early-life risk factors for Alzheimer disease. *Alzheimer Disease & Associated Disorders,* *20*(1), 63-72. doi:10.1097/01.wad.0000201854.62116.d7

Cannon-Albright, L. A., Foster, N. L., Schliep, K., Farnham, J. M., Teerlink, C. C., Kaddas, H., . . . Kauwe, J. S. K. (2019). Relative risk for Alzheimer disease based on complete family history. *Neurology,* *92*(15), e1745-e1753. doi:10.1212/WNL.0000000000007231

Carvalho, D. Z., St Louis, E. K., Knopman, D. S., Boeve, B. F., Lowe, V. J., Roberts, R. O., . . . Vemuri, P. (2018). Association of excessive daytime sleepiness with longitudinal beta-amyloid accumulation in elderly persons without dementia. *JAMA Neurology, 75*(6), 672-680. doi:10.1001/jamaneurol.2018.0049

Cryan, J. F., & Dinan, T. G. (2012). Mind-altering microorganisms: the impact of the gut microbiota on brain and behaviour. *Nature Reviews Neuroscience, 13*(10), 701-712. doi:10.1038/nrn3346

Daviglus, M. L., Plassman, B. L., Pirzada, A., Bell, C. C., Bowen, P. E., Burke, J. R., . . . Williams, J. W., Jr. (2011). Risk factors and preventive interventions for Alzheimer disease: state of the science. *Archives of Neurology, 68*(9), 1185-1190. doi:10.1001/archneurol.2011.100

Diniz, B. S., Butters, M. A., Albert, S. M., Dew, M. A., & Reynolds, C. F., 3rd. (2013). Late-life depression and risk of vascular dementia and Alzheimer's disease: Systematic review and meta-analysis of community-based cohort studies. *The British Journal of Psychiatry, 202*(5), 329-335. doi:10.1192/bjp.bp.112.118307

Donovan, N. J., Locascio, J. J., Marshall, G. A., Gatchel, J., Hanseeuw, B. J., Rentz, D. M., . . . Harvard Aging Brain, S. (2018). Longitudinal association of amyloid beta and anxious-depressive symptoms in cognitively normal older adults. *American Journal of Psychiatry, 175*(6), 530-537. doi:10.1176/appi.ajp.2017.17040442

Ewers, M., Insel, P. S., Stern, Y., Weiner, M. W., & Alzheimer's Disease Neuroimaging, I. (2013). Cognitive reserve associated with FDG-PET in preclinical Alzheimer disease. *Neurology, 80*(13), 1194-1201. doi:10.1212/WNL.0b013e31828970c2

Fotenos, A. F., Mintun, M. A., Snyder, A. Z., Morris, J. C., & Buckner, R. L. (2008). Brain volume decline in aging: Evidence for a relation between socioeconomic status, preclinical Alzheimer disease, and reserve. *Archives of Neurology, 65*(1), 113-120. doi:10.1001/archneurol.2007.27

Frederiksen, K. S., Gjerum, L., Waldemar, G., & Hasselbalch, S. G. (2019). Physical activity as a moderator of Alzheimer pathology:

Reference

A systematic review of observational studies. *Current Alzheimer's Research*. doi:10.2174/1567205016666190315095151

Gallaway, P. J., Miyake, H., Buchowski, M. S., Shimada, M., Yoshitake, Y., Kim, A. S., & Hongu, N. (2017). Physical activity: A viable way to reduce the risks of mild cognitive impairment, Alzheimer's disease, and vascular dementia in older adults. *Brain Sciences, 7*(2). doi:10.3390/brainsci7020022

Geda, Y. E., Roberts, R. O., Mielke, M. M., Knopman, D. S., Christianson, T. J., Pankratz, V. S., . . . Rocca, W. A. (2014). Baseline neuropsychiatric symptoms and the risk of incident mild cognitive impairment: A population-based study. *American Journal of Psychiatry, 171*(5), 572-581. doi:10.1176/appi.ajp.2014.13060821

Groot, C., van Loenhoud, A. C., Barkhof, F., van Berckel, B. N. M., Koene, T., Teunissen, C. C., . . . Ossenkoppele, R. (2018). Differential effects of cognitive reserve and brain reserve on cognition in Alzheimer disease. *Neurology, 90*(2), e149-e156. doi:10.1212/WNL.0000000000004802

Halloway, S., Arfanakis, K., Wilbur, J., Schoeny, M. E., & Pressler, S. J. (2018). Accelerometer physical activity is associated with greater gray matter volumes in older adults without dementia or mild cognitive impairment. The *Journals of Gerontology, Series B: Psychological Sciences and Social Sciences*. doi:10.1093/geronb/gby010

Hazar, N., Seddigh, L., Rampisheh, Z., & Nojomi, M. (2016). Population attributable fraction of modifiable risk factors for Alzheimer disease: A systematic review of systematic reviews. *Iranian Journal of Neurology, 15*(3), 164-172.

Hickman, R. A., Faustin, A., & Wisniewski, T. (2016). Alzheimer disease and its growing epidemic: Risk factors, biomarkers, and the urgent need for therapeutics. *Neurologic Clinics, 34*(4), 941-953. doi:10.1016/j.ncl.2016.06.009

Ju, Y. E., Lucey, B. P., & Holtzman, D. M. (2014). Sleep and Alzheimer disease pathology—a bidirectional relationship. *Nature Reviews Neurology, 10*(2), 115-119. doi:10.1038/nrneurol.2013.269

Kabeshita, Y., Adachi, H., Matsushita, M., Kanemoto, H., Sato, S., Suzuki, Y., . . . Kazui, H. (2017). Sleep disturbances are key symptoms of very early stage Alzheimer disease with behavioral and psychological symptoms: A Japan multi-center cross-sectional study (J-BIRD). *International Journal of Geriatric Psychiatry, 32*(2), 222-230. doi:10.1002/gps.4470

Ko, K., Byun, M. S., Yi, D., Lee, J. H., Kim, C. H., & Lee, D. Y. (2018). Early-life cognitive activity is related to reduced neurodegeneration in Alzheimer signature regions in late life. *Frontiers in Aging Neuroscience, 10,* 70. doi:10.3389/fnagi.2018.00070

Litwin, H., & Stoeckel, K. J. (2016). Social network, activity participation, and cognition: A complex relationship. *Research on Aging, 38*(1), 76-97. doi:10.1177/0164027515581422

Luchsinger, J. A., & Mayeux, R. (2004). Dietary factors and Alzheimer's disease. *Lancet Neurology, 3*(10), 579-587. doi:10.1016/S1474-4422(04)00878-6

Muller, S., Preische, O., Sohrabi, H. R., Graber, S., Jucker, M., Ringman, J. M., . . . Dominantly Inherited Alzheimer, N. (2018). Relationship between physical activity, cognition, and Alzheimer pathology in autosomal dominant Alzheimer's disease. *Alzheimer's & Dementia, 14*(11), 1427-1437. doi:10.1016/j.jalz.2018.06.3059

Musiek, E. S., Xiong, D. D., & Holtzman, D. M. (2015). Sleep, circadian rhythms, and the pathogenesis of Alzheimer disease.

Experimental & Molecular Medicine, 47, e148. doi:10.1038/emm.2014.121

Neu, S. C., Pa, J., Kukull, W., Beekly, D., Kuzma, A., Gangadharan, P., . . . Toga, A. W. (2017). Apolipoprotein E genotype and sex risk factors for Alzheimer disease: A meta-analysis. *JAMA Neurology,* 74(10), 1178-1189. doi:10.1001/jamaneurol.2017.2188

Ngandu, T., Lehtisalo, J., Solomon, A., Levalahti, E., Ahtiluoto, S., Antikainen, R., . . . Kivipelto, M. (2015). A 2 year multidomain intervention of diet, exercise, cognitive training, and vascular risk monitoring versus control to prevent cognitive decline in at-risk elderly people (FINGER): A randomised controlled trial. *Lancet, 385*(9984), 2255-2263. doi:10.1016/S0140-6736(15)60461-5

Saez de Asteasu, M. L., Martinez-Velilla, N., Zambom-Ferraresi, F., Casas-Herrero, A., & Izquierdo, M. (2017). Role of physical exercise on cognitive function in healthy older adults: A systematic review of randomized clinical trials. *Ageing Research Reviews, 37,* 117-134. doi:10.1016/j.arr.2017.05.007

Sato, N., & Morishita, R. (2013). Roles of vascular and metabolic components in cognitive dysfunction of Alzheimer disease: Short- and long-term modification by non-genetic risk factors. *Frontiers in Aging Neuroscience, 5,* 64. doi:10.3389/fnagi.2013.00064

Shah, R. (2013). The role of nutrition and diet in Alzheimer disease: a systematic review. *Journal of the American Medical Directors Association, 14*(6), 398-402. doi:10.1016/j.jamda.2013.01.014

Takatori, S., Wang, W., Iguchi, A., & Tomita, T. (2019). Genetic risk factors for Alzheimer disease: Emerging roles of microglia in disease pathomechanisms. *Advances in Experimental Medicine and Biology, 1118,* 83-116. doi:10.1007/978-3-030-05542-4_5

van Paasschen, J., Clare, L., Yuen, K. S., Woods, R. T., Evans, S. J., Parkinson, C. H., . . . Linden, D. E. (2013). Cognitive rehabilitation changes memory-related brain activity in people with Alzheimer disease. *Neurorehabilitation and Neural Repair, 27*(5), 448-459. doi:10.1177/1545968312471902

Wengreen, H., Munger, R. G., Cutler, A., Quach, A., Bowles, A., Corcoran, C., . . . Welsh-Bohmer, K. A. (2013). Prospective study of Dietary Approaches to Stop Hypertension- and Mediterranean-style dietary patterns and age-related cognitive change: The Cache County Study on Memory, Health and Aging. *The American Journal of Clinical Nutrition, 98*(5), 1263-1271. doi:10.3945/ajcn.112.051276

World Health, O. (2018). Risk reduction of cognitive decline and dementia. Retrieved from https://www.who.int/mental_health/neurology/dementia/guidelin es_risk_reduction/en/

Chapter 4

American College of Sports Medicine. (2018). *ACSM's Guidelines for Exercise Testing and Prescription 10th Edition*. Philadelphia, PA: Wolters Kluwer.

American College of Sports Medicine position stand. Progression models in resistance training for healthy adults. (2009). *Medicine & Science in Sports & Exercise, 41*(3), 687-708. doi:10.1249/MSS.0b013e3181915670

Bassett, D. R., Jr., & Howley, E. T. (2000). Limiting factors for maximum oxygen uptake and determinants of endurance performance. *Medicine & Science in Sports & Exercise, 32*(1), 70-84.

Blair, S. N., Kampert, J. B., Kohl, H. W., 3rd, Barlow, C. E., Macera, C. A., Paffenbarger, R. S., Jr., & Gibbons, L. W. (1996). Influences of cardiorespiratory fitness and other precursors on cardiovascular disease and all-cause mortality in men and women. *The Journal of the American Medical Association,* *276*(3), 205-210.

Bouchard, C., & Rankinen, T. (2001). Individual differences in response to regular physical activity. *Medicine & Science in Sports and Exercise, 33*(6 Suppl), S446-451; discussion S452-443.

Bronas, U.G., & Salisbury, D.L.. (2014). Clinical strategies for managing dyslipidemia. *American Journal of Lifestyle Medicine, 8*(4), 216-230.

Centers for Disease Control and Prevention (2018). Cholesterol fact sheet. Retrieved from https://www.cdc.gov/dhdsp/data_statistics/fact_sheets/fs_cholesterol.htm

Centers for Disease Control and Prevention. (2018). High blood pressure fact sheet. Retrieved from https://www.cdc.gov/dhdsp/data_statistics/fact_sheets/fs_blood pressure.htm

Colberg, S. R., Sigal, R. J., Yardley, J. E., Riddell, M. C., Dunstan, D. W., Dempsey, P. C., . . . Tate, D. F. (2016). Physical activity/exercise and diabetes: A position statement of the American Diabetes Association. *Diabetes Care, 39*(11), 2065-2079. doi:10.2337/dc16-1728

Garber, C. E., Blissmer, B., Deschenes, M. R., Franklin, B. A., Lamonte, M. J., Lee, I. M., . . . American College of Sports, M. (2011). American College of Sports Medicine position stand. Quantity and quality of exercise for developing and maintaining cardiorespiratory, musculoskeletal, and neuromotor fitness in apparently healthy adults: guidance for prescribing exercise. *Medicine & Science in Sports & Exercise, 43*(7), 1334-1359. doi:10.1249/MSS.0b013e318213fefb

Kohrt, W. M., Bloomfield, S. A., Little, K. D., Nelson, M. E., & Yingling, V. R. (2004). American College of Sports Medicine

Position Stand: Physical activity and bone health. *Medicine & Science in Sports & Exercise, 36*(11), 1985-1996.

Lee, D. C., Sui, X., Ortega, F. B., Kim, Y. S., Church, T. S., Winett, R. A., . . . Blair, S. N. (2011). Comparisons of leisure-time physical activity and cardiorespiratory fitness as predictors of all-cause mortality in men and women. *The British Journal of Sports Medicine, 45*(6), 504-510. doi:10.1136/bjsm.2009.066209

Leon A.S., & Bronas U.G. (2009). Dyslipidemia and risk of coronary artery disease: Role of lifestyle approaches for its management. *American Journal of Lifestyle Medicine, 3*(4), 257-273.

Pescatello, L. S., MacDonald, H. V., Lamberti, L., & Johnson, B. T. (2015). Exercise for hypertension: A prescription update integrating existing recommendations with emerging research. *Current Hypertension Reports, 17*(11), 87. doi:10.1007/s11906-015-0600-y

Santos, C. Y., Snyder, P. J., Wu, W. C., Zhang, M., Echeverria, A., & Alber, J. (2017). Pathophysiologic relationship between Alzheimer's disease, cerebrovascular disease, and cardiovascular risk: A review and synthesis. *Alzheimer's & Dementia (Amst), 7*, 69-87. doi:10.1016/j.dadm.2017.01.005

Stampfer, M. J. (2006). Cardiovascular disease and Alzheimer's disease: common links. *Journal of Internal Medicine, 260*(3), 211-223. doi:10.1111/j.1365-2796.2006.01687.x

U.S. Department of Health and Human Services, P. A. A. C. (2018). *Physical activity guidelines advisory committee scientific report.* Washington DC Retrieved from https://health.gov/paguidelines/second-edition/report/

Musich, S., Wang, S. S., Hawkins, K., & Greame, C. (2017). The frequency and health benefits of physical activity for older adults. *Population Health Management, 20*(3), 199-207. doi:10.1089/pop.2016.0071

Reference

Nelson, M. E., Rejeski, W. J., Blair, S. N., Duncan, P. W., Judge, J. O., King, A. C., . . . Castaneda-Sceppa, C. (2007). Physical activity and public health in older adults: recommendation from the American College of Sports Medicine and the American Heart Association. *Medicine & Science in Sports & Exercise, 39*(8), 1435-1445. doi:10.1249/mss.0b013e3180616aa2

Pescatello, L. S., MacDonald, H. V., Lamberti, L., & Johnson, B. T. (2015). Exercise for hypertension: A prescription update integrating existing recommendations with emerging research. *Current Hypertension Reports, 17*(11), 87. doi:10.1007/s11906-015-0600-y

Santos, C. Y., Snyder, P. J., Wu, W. C., Zhang, M., Echeverria, A., & Alber, J. (2017). Pathophysiologic relationship between Alzheimer's disease, cerebrovascular disease, and cardiovascular risk: A review and synthesis. *Alzheimer's & Dementia (Amst), 7*, 69-87. doi:10.1016/j.dadm.2017.01.005

Siddarth, D., Siddarth, P., & Lavretsky, H. (2014). An observational study of the health benefits of yoga or tai chi compared with aerobic exercise in community-dwelling middle-aged and older adults. *American Journal of Geriatric Psychiatry, 22*(3), 272-273. doi:10.1016/j.jagp.2013.01.065

Sparling, P. B., Howard, B. J., Dunstan, D. W., & Owen, N. (2015). Recommendations for physical activity in older adults. *BMJ, 350*, h100. doi:10.1136/bmj.h100

Stamatakis, E., Gale, J., Bauman, A., Ekelund, U., Hamer, M., & Ding, D. (2019). Sitting time, physical activity, and risk of mortality in adults. *Journal of the American College of Cardiology, 73*(16), 2062-2072. doi:10.1016/j.jacc.2019.02.031

Stampfer, M. J. (2006). Cardiovascular disease and Alzheimer's disease: common links. *Journal of Internal Medicine, 260*(3), 211-223. doi:10.1111/j.1365-2796.2006.01687.x

Taylor, A. H., Cable, N. T., Faulkner, G., Hillsdon, M.,

Narici, M., & Van Der Bij, A. K. (2004). Physical activity and older adults: A review of health benefits and the effectiveness of interventions. *Journal of Sports Sciences, 22*(8), 703-725. doi:10.1080/02640410410001712421.

U.S. Department of Health and Human Services, P. A. A. C. (2018). *Physical Activity Guidelines Advisory Committee Scientific Report.* Washington DC Retrieved from https://health.gov/paguidelines/second-edition/report/

Chapter 5

Allendorfer, J. B., & Arida, R. M. (2018). Role of physical activity and exercise in alleviating cognitive impairment in people with epilepsy. *Clinical Therapeutics, 40*(1), 26-34. doi:10.1016/j.clinthera.2017.12.004

Azimi, M., Gharakhanlou, R., Naghdi, N., Khodadadi, D., & Heysieattalab, S. (2018). Moderate treadmill exercise ameliorates amyloid-beta-induced learning and memory impairment, possibly via increasing AMPK activity and up-regulation of the PGC-1alpha/FNDC5/BDNF pathway. *Peptides, 102*, 78-88. doi:10.1016/j.peptides.2017.12.027

Brenes, G. A., Sohl, S., Wells, R. E., Befus, D., Campos, C. L., & Danhauer, S. C. (2019). The effects of yoga on patients with mild cognitive impairment and dementia: A scoping review. *American Journal of Geriatric Psychiatry, 27*(2), 188-197. doi:10.1016/j.jagp.2018.10.013

Bronas, U. G., Salisbury, D., Kelly, K., Leon, A., Chow, L., & Yu, F. (2017). Determination of aerobic capacity via cycle ergometer exercise testing in Alzheimer's disease. *American Journal of Alzheimer's Disease and Other Dementias, 32*(8), 500-508. doi:10.1177/1533317517720065

Reference

Colcombe, S., & Kramer, A. F. (2003). Fitness effects on the cognitive function of older adults: A meta-analytic study. *Psychological Science, 14*(2), 125-130.

Cotman, C. W., & Berchtold, N. C. (2007). Physical activity and the maintenance of cognition: Learning from animal models. *Alzheimer's & Dementia, 3*(2), S30-S37.

Davis, J. C., Bryan, S., Marra, C. A., Sharma, D., Chan, A., Beattie, B. L., . . . Liu-Ambrose, T. (2013). An economic evaluation of resistance training and aerobic training versus balance and toning exercises in older adults with mild cognitive impairment. *PloS one, 8*(5), e63031. doi:10.1371/journal.pone.0063031

Eggermont, L., Swaab, D., Luiten, P., & Scherder, E. (2006). Exercise, cognition and Alzheimer's disease: more is not necessarily better. *Neuroscience & Biobehaval Reviews, 30*(4), 562-575. doi:10.1016/j.neubiorev.2005.10.004

Epperly, T., Dunay, M. A., & Boice, J. L. (2017). Alzheimer disease: Pharmacologic and nonpharmacologic therapies for cognitive and functional symptoms. *American Family Physician, 95*(12), 771-778.

Erickson, K. I., & Kramer, A. F. (2009). Aerobic exercise effects on cognitive and neural plasticity in older adults. *The British Journal of Sports Medicine, 43*(1), 22-24.

Etnier, J. L., Nowell, P. M., Landers, D. M., & Sibley, B. A. (2006). A meta-regression to examine the relationship between aerobic fitness and cognitive performance. *Brain Research Reviews, 52*(1), 119-130.

Fahimi, A., Baktir, M. A., Moghadam, S., Mojabi, F. S., Sumanth, K., McNerney, M. W., . . . Salehi, A. (2017). Physical exercise induces structural alterations in the hippocampal astrocytes: exploring the role of BDNF-TrkB signaling. *Brain Structure and Function, 222*(4), 1797-1808. doi:10.1007/s00429-016-1308-8

Farhang, M., Miranda-Castillo, C., Rubio, M., & Furtado, G. (2019). Impact of mind-body interventions in older adults with mild cognitive impairment: A systematic review. *International Psychogeriatrics*, 1-24. doi:10.1017/S1041610218002302

Fiatarone Singh, M. A., Gates, N., Saigal, N., Wilson, G. C., Meiklejohn, J., Brodaty, H., . . . Valenzuela, M. (2014). The Study of Mental and Resistance Training (SMART) study-resistance training and/or cognitive training in mild cognitive impairment: A randomized, double-blind, double-sham controlled trial. *Journal of the American Medical Directors Association, 15*(12), 873-880. doi:10.1016/j.jamda.2014.09.010

Fogarty, J. N., Murphy, K. J., McFarlane, B., Montero-Odasso, M., Wells, J., Troyer, A. K., . . . Hansen, K. T. (2016). Taoist tai chi(R) and memory intervention for individuals with mild cognitive impairment. *Journal of Aging and Physical Activity, 24*(2), 169-180. doi:10.1123/japa.2014-0062

Gothe, N. P., & McAuley, E. (2015). Yoga and cognition: A meta-analysis of chronic and acute effects. *Psychosomatic Medicine, 77*(7), 784-797. doi:10.1097/PSY.0000000000000218

Guure, C. B., Ibrahim, N. A., Adam, M. B., & Said, S. M. (2017). Impact of physical activity on cognitive decline, dementia, and its subtypes: Meta-analysis of prospective studies. *BioMed Research International, 2017*, 9016924. doi:https://dx.doi.org/10.1155/2017/9016924

Intlekofer, K. A., & Cotman, C. W. (2013). Exercise counteracts declining hippocampal function in aging and Alzheimer's disease. *Neurobiology Disease, 57*, 47-55. doi:10.1016/j.nbd.2012.06.011

Jensen, C. S., Bahl, J. M., Ostergaard, L. B., Hogh, P., Wermuth, L., Heslegrave, A., . . . Simonsen, A. H. (2019). Exercise as a potential modulator of inflammation in patients with Alzheimer's disease measured in cerebrospinal fluid and plasma.

Experimental Gerontology, 121, 91-98. doi:10.1016/j.exger.2019.04.003

Jensen, C. S., Simonsen, A. H., Siersma, V., Beyer, N., Frederiksen, K. S., Gottrup, H., . . . Hasselbalch, S. G. (2019). Patients with Alzheimer's disease who carry the APOE epsilon4 allele benefit more from physical exercise. *Alzheimer's & Dementia, 5,* 99-106. doi:10.1016/j.trci.2019.02.007

Lam, L. C., Chau, R. C., Wong, B. M., Fung, A. W., Tam, C. W., Leung, G. T., . . . Chan, W. M. (2012). A 1-year randomized controlled trial comparing mind body exercise (tai chi) with stretching and toning exercise on cognitive function in older Chinese adults at risk of cognitive decline. *Journal of the American Medical Directors Association, 13*(6), 568 e515-520. doi:10.1016/j.jamda.2012.03.008

Lamb, S. E., Mistry, D., Alleyne, S., Atherton, N., Brown, D., Copsey, B., . . . Sheehan, B. (2018). Aerobic and strength training exercise programme for cognitive impairment in people with mild to moderate dementia: The DAPA RCT. *Health Technology Assess, 22*(28), 1-202. doi:10.3310/hta22280

Li, M. Y., Huang, M. M., Li, S. Z., Tao, J., Zheng, G. H., & Chen, L. D. (2017). The effects of aerobic exercise on the structure and function of DMN-related brain regions: A systematic review. *International Journal of Neuroscience, 127*(7), 634-649. doi:10.1080/00207454.2016.1212855

Marston, K. J., Brown, B. M., Rainey-Smith, S. R., & Peiffer, J. J. (2019). Resistance exercise-induced responses in physiological factors linked with cognitive health. *Journal of Alzheimer's Disease, 68*(1), 39-64. doi:10.3233/JAD-181079

Mavros, Y., Gates, N., Wilson, G. C., Jain, N., Meiklejohn, J., Brodaty, H., . . . Fiatarone Singh, M. A. (2017). Mediation of cognitive function improvements by strength gains after resistance training in older adults with mild cognitive impairment:

Outcomes of the study of mental and resistance training. *Journal of the American Geriatrics Society, 65*(3), 550-559. doi:10.1111/jgs.14542

Nagamatsu, L. S., Handy, T. C., Hsu, C. L., Voss, M., & Liu-Ambrose, T. (2012). Resistance training promotes cognitive and functional brain plasticity in seniors with probable mild cognitive impairment. *Archives of Internal Medicine, 172*(8), 666-668. doi:10.1001/archinternmed.2012.379

Northey, J. M., Cherbuin, N., Pumpa, K. L., Smee, D. J., & Rattray, B. (2018). Exercise interventions for cognitive function in adults older than 50: A systematic review with meta-analysis. *British Journal of Sports Medicine, 52*(3), 154-160. doi:10.1136/bjsports-2016-096587

Panza, G. A., Taylor, B. A., MacDonald, H. V., Johnson, B. T., Zaleski, A. L., Livingston, J., . . . Pescatello, L. S. (2018). Can exercise improve cognitive symptoms of Alzheimer's disease? A meta-analysis. *Journal of the American Geriatrics Society, 66*(3), 489-495. doi:https://dx.doi.org/10.1111/jgs.15241

Robitaille, A., Muniz, G., Lindwall, M., Piccinin, A. M., Hoffman, L., Johansson, B., & Hofer, S. M. (2014). Physical activity and cognitive functioning in the oldest old: Within- and between-person cognitive activity and psychosocial mediators. *European Journal of Ageing, 11*(4), 333-347. doi:10.1007/s10433-014-0314-z

Saez de Asteasu, M. L., Martinez-Velilla, N., Zambom-Ferraresi, F., Casas-Herrero, A., & Izquierdo, M. (2017). Role of physical exercise on cognitive function in healthy older adults: A systematic review of randomized clinical trials. *Ageing Research Reviews, 37*, 117-134. doi:10.1016/j.arr.2017.05.007

Salisbury, D., Yu, F. (2018). Aerobic fitness and cognitive changes after exercise training in Alzheimer's disease. *Journal of Exercise and Clinical Psychology, 6*(2), 22-28.

Reference

Sanders, L. M. J., Hortobagyi, T., la Bastide-van Gemert, S., van der Zee, E. A., & van Heuvelen, M. J. G. (2019). Dose-response relationship between exercise and cognitive function in older adults with and without cognitive impairment: A systematic review and meta-analysis. *PloS one, 14*(1), e0210036. doi:10.1371/journal.pone.0210036

Santos-Lozano, A., Pareja-Galeano, H., Sanchis-Gomar, F., Quindos-Rubial, M., Fiuza-Luces, C., Cristi-Montero, C., . . . Lucia, A. (2016). Physical activity and Alzheimer disease: A protective association. *Mayo Clinic proceedings, 91*(8), 999-1020. doi:https://dx.doi.org/10.1016/j.mayocp.2016.04.024

Sungkarat, S., Boripuntakul, S., Chattipakorn, N., Watcharasaksilp, K., & Lord, S. R. (2017). Effects of tai chi on cognition and fall risk in older adults with mild cognitive impairment: A randomized controlled trial. *Journal of the American Geriatrics Society, 65*(4), 721-727. doi:10.1111/jgs.14594

Tari, A. R., Norevik, C. S., Scrimgeour, N. R., Kobro-Flatmoen, A., Storm-Mathisen, J., Bergersen, L. H., . . . Wisloff, U. (2019). Are the neuroprotective effects of exercise training systemically mediated? *Progress in Cardiovascular Diseases, 62*(2), 94-101. doi:10.1016/j.pcad.2019.02.003

van der Kleij, L. A., Petersen, E. T., Siebner, H. R., Hendrikse, J., Frederiksen, K. S., Sobol, N. A., . . . Garde, E. (2018). The effect of physical exercise on cerebral blood flow in Alzheimer's disease. *NeuroImage Clinical, 20,* 650-654. doi:10.1016/j.nicl.2018.09.003

Vilela, T. C., Effting, P. S., Dos Santos Pedroso, G., Farias, H., Paganini, L., Rebelo Sorato, H., . . . de Pinho, R. A. (2018). Aerobic and strength training induce changes in oxidative stress parameters and elicit modifications of various cellular components in skeletal muscle of aged rats. *Experimental Gerontology, 106*, 21-27. doi:10.1016/j.exger.2018.02.014

Wayne, P. M., Walsh, J. N., Taylor-Piliae, R. E., Wells, R. E., Papp, K. V., Donovan, N. J., & Yeh, G. Y. (2014). Effect of tai chi on cognitive performance in older adults: systematic review and meta-analysis. *Journal of the American Geriatrics Society, 62*(1), 25-39. doi:10.1111/jgs.12611

Wilke, J., Giesche, F., Klier, K., Vogt, L., Herrmann, E., & Banzer, W. (2019). Acute effects of resistance exercise on cognitive function in healthy adults: A systematic review with multilevel meta-analysis. *Sports Medicine.* doi:10.1007/s40279-019-01085-x

Yoon, D. H., Kang, D., Kim, H. J., Kim, J. S., Song, H. S., & Song, W. (2017). Effect of elastic band-based high-speed power training on cognitive function, physical performance and muscle strength in older women with mild cognitive impairment. *Geriatrics & Gerontology International, 17*(5), 765-772. doi:10.1111/ggi.12784

Yu, F. (2011). Guiding research and practice: A conceptual model for aerobic exercise training in Alzheimer's disease. *American Journal of Alzheimers Disease and Other Dementias, 26*(3), 184-194. doi:10.1177/1533317511402317

Yu, F., Bronas, U. G., Konety, S., Nelson, N. W., Dysken, M., Jack, C., Jr., . . . Smith, G. (2014). Effects of aerobic exercise on cognition and hippocampal volume in Alzheimer's disease: study protocol of a randomized controlled trial (The FIT-AD™ trial). *Trials, 15*, 394. doi:10.1186/1745-6215-15-394 1745-6215-15-394 [pii]

Yu, F., Nelson, N. W., Savik, K., Wyman, J. F., Dysken, M., & Bronas, U. G. (2013). Affecting cognition and quality of life via aerobic exercise in Alzheimer's disease. *Western Journal of Nursing Research, 35*(1), 24-38. doi:10.1177/0193945911420174

Yu, F., Thomas, W., Nelson, N. W., Bronas, U. G., Dysken, M., & Wyman, J. (2015). Impact of a 6-month aerobic exercise on Alzheimer's symptoms. *Journal of Applied Gerontology, 34*(4), 484-500.

Chapter 6

American Geriatrics Society Expert Panel on the Care of Older Adults with Multimorbidity. (2012). Patient-centered care for older adults with multiple chronic conditions: A stepwise approach from the American Geriatrics Society: American Geriatrics Society expert panel on the care of older adults with multimorbidity. *Journal of the American Geriatrics Society, 60*(10), 1957-1968.

Bayles, K. A., Tomoeda, C. K., Cruz, R. F., & Mahendra, N. (2000). Communication abilities of individuals with late-stage Alzheimer disease. *Alzheimer Disease & Associated Disorders, 14*(3), 176-181.

Bergman, M., Graff, C., Eriksdotter, M., Fugl-Meyer, K. S., & Schuster, M. (2016). The meaning of living close to a person with Alzheimer disease. *Medicine, Health Care and Philosophy, 19*(3), 341-349. doi:10.1007/s11019-016-9696-3

Bossen, A. L., Specht, J. K., & McKenzie, S. E. (2009). Needs of people with early-stage Alzheimer's disease: reviewing the evidence. *Journal of Gerontological Nursing, 35*(3), 8-15.

Brownie, S., & Nancarrow, S. (2013). Effects of person-centered care on residents and staff in aged-care facilities: a systematic review. *Clinical Interventions in Aging, 8*, 1-10. doi:10.2147/CIA.S38589

Chenoweth, L., Stein-Parbury, J., Lapkin, S., Wang, A., Liu, Z., & Williams, A. (2019). Effects of person-centered care at the organisational-level for people with dementia. A systematic review. *PloS one, 14*(2), e0212686. doi:10.1371/journal.pone.0212686

Cott, C. A., Dawson, P., Sidani, S., & Wells, D. (2002). The effects of a walking/talking program on communication, ambulation, and functional status in residents with Alzheimer disease. *Alzheimer Disease & Associated Disorders, 16*(2), 81-87.

de Carvalho, I. A., & Mansur, L. L. (2008). Validation of ASHA FACS-functional assessment of communication skills for Alzheimer disease population. *Alzheimer Disease & Associated Disorders, 22*(4), 375-381.

Hakansson Eklund, J., Holmstrom, I. K., Kumlin, T., Kaminsky, E., Skoglund, K., Hoglander, J., . . . Summer Meranius, M. (2019). "Same same or different?" A review of reviews of person-centered and patient-centered care. *Patient Education and Counseling, 102*(1), 3-11. doi:10.1016/j.pec.2018.08.029

Karlsson, E., Savenstedt, S., Axelsson, K., Zingmark, K. (2014). Stories about life narrated by people with Alzheimer's disease. *Journal of Advanced Nursing, 70*(12), 2791-2799. doi:doi: 10.1111/jan.12429

Li, J., & Porock, D. (2014). Resident outcomes of person-centered care in long-term care: A narrative review of interventional research. *International Journal of Nursing Studies, 51*(10), 1395-1415. doi:10.1016/j.ijnurstu.2014.04.003

Morello, A., Lima, T. M., & Brandao, L. (2017). Language and communication non-pharmacological interventions in patients with Alzheimer's disease: a systematic review. Communication intervention in Alzheimer. *Dementia & Neuropsychologia, 11*(3), 227-241. doi:10.1590/1980-57642016dn11-030004

Penrod, J., Yu, F., Kolanowski, A., Fick, D. M., Loeb, S. J., & Hupcey, J. E. (2007). Reframing person-centered nursing care for persons with dementia. *Research and Theory for Nursing Practice, 21*(1), 57-72.

Reisberg, B., Shao, Y., Golomb, J., Monteiro, I., Torossian, C., Boksay, I., . . . Kenowsky, S. (2017). Comprehensive, individualized, person-centered management of community-residing persons with moderate-to-severe Alzheimer disease: A randomized controlled trial. *Dementia and Geriatric Cognitive Disorders, 43*(1-2), 100-117. doi:10.1159/000455397

Rodriguez-Rodriguez, A., Martel-Monagas, L., & Lopez-Rodriguez, A. (2010). Enhancing the communication flow between Alzheimer patients, caregivers, and neuropsychologists. *Advances in Experimental Medicine and Biology, 680*, 601-607. doi:10.1007/978-1-4419-5913-3_66

Small, J. A., & Gutman, G. (2002). Recommended and reported use of communication strategies in Alzheimer caregiving. *Alzheimer Disease & Associated Disorders, 16*(4), 270-278.

Yun, D., & Choi, J. (2019). Person-centered rehabilitation care and outcomes: A systematic literature review. *International Journal of Nursing Studies, 93*, 74-83. doi:10.1016/j.ijnurstu.2019.02.012

Chapter 7

American College of Sports Medicine (2018). *ACSM's Guidelines for Exercise Testing and Prescription 10th Edition*. Philadelphia, PA: Wolters Kluwer.

Bethancourt, H. J., Rosenberg, D. E., Beatty, T., & Arterburn, D. E. (2014). Barriers to and facilitators of physical activity program use among older adults. *Clinical Medicine & Research, 12*(1-2), 10-20. doi:10.3121/cmr.2013.1171

Borg, G. (1998). *Borg's Perceived Exertion and Pain Scales*. Champaign, IL: Human Kinetics.

Bronas, U. G., Salisbury, D., Kelly, K., Leon, A., Chow, L., & Yu, F. (2017). Determination of aerobic capacity via cycle ergometer exercise testing in Alzheimer's disease. *American Journal of Alzheimer's Disease and Other Dementias, 32*(8), 500-508. doi:10.1177/1533317517720065

Fletcher, G. F., Ades, P. A., Kligfield, P., Arena, R., Balady, G. J., Bittner, V. A., . . . Williams, M. A. (2013). Exercise standards for testing and training: A scientific statement from the American Heart Association. *Circulation, 128*(8), 873-934. doi:10.1161/CIR.0b013e31829b5b44

Garber, C. E., Blissmer, B., Deschenes, M. R., Franklin, B. A., Lamonte, M. J., Lee, I. M., . . . American College of Sports, M. (2011). American College of Sports Medicine position stand. Quantity and quality of exercise for developing and maintaining cardiorespiratory, musculoskeletal, and neuromotor fitness in apparently healthy adults: guidance for prescribing exercise. *Medicine & Science in Sports & Exercise, 43*(7), 1334-1359. doi:10.1249/MSS.0b013e318213fefb

Kreatsoulas, C., Shannon, H. S., Giacomini, M., Velianou, J. L., & Anand, S. S. (2013). Reconstructing angina: Cardiac symptoms are the same in women and men. In *JAMA Internal Medicine* (Vol. 173, pp. 829-831).

Laboratories, A. T. S. C. o. P. S. f. C. P. F. (2002). ATS statement: guidelines for the six-minute walk test. *American Journal of Respiratory & Critical Care Medicine, 166*(1), 111-117.

Panza, G. A., Taylor, B. A., MacDonald, H. V., Johnson, B. T., Zaleski, A. L., Livingston, J., . . . Pescatello, L. S. (2018). Can exercise improve cognitive symptoms of Alzheimer's disease? *Journal of the American Geriatrics Society, 66*(3), 487-495. doi:10.1111/jgs.15241

Reed, J. L., & Pipe, A. L. (2014). The talk test: a useful tool for prescribing and monitoring exercise intensity. *Current Opinion in Cardiology, 29*(5), 475-480. doi:10.1097/hco.0000000000000097

Resnick, B., Ory, M. G., Hora, K., Rogers, M. E., Page, P., Bolin, J. N., . . . Bazzarre, T. L. (2008). A proposal for a new screening paradigm and tool called Exercise Assessment and Screening for You (EASY). *Journal of Aging and Physical Activity, 16*(2), 215-233.

Riebe, D., Franklin, B. A., Thompson, P. D., Garber, C. E., Whitfield, G. P., Magal, M., & Pescatello, L. S. (2015). Updating ACSM's recommendations for exercise preparticipation health screening. *Medicine & Science in Sports & Exercise, 47*(11), 2473-2479. doi:10.1249/mss.0000000000000664

Singh, S. J., Morgan, M. D., Scott, S., Walters, D., & Hardman, A. E. (1992). Development of a shuttle walking test of disability in patients with chronic airways obstruction. *Thorax, 47*(12), 1019-1024.

World Health Organization. (2019). Global Strategy on Diet, Physical Activity, and Health. Retrieved from https://www.who.int/dietphysicalactivity/factsheet_adults/en/

Chapter 8

Benjamin, E. J., Blaha, M. J., Chiuve, S. E., Cushman, M., Das, S. R., Deo, R., . . . Muntner, P. (2017). Heart disease and stroke statistics-2017 update: A report from the American Heart Association. *Circulation, 135*(10), e146-e603. doi:10.1161/cir.0000000000000485

Borg, G. (1998). *Borg's Perceived Exertion and Pain Scales.* Champaign, IL: Human Kinetics.

Centers for Disease Control and Prevention. (2017). New CDC report: More than 100 million Americans have diabetes or prediabetes. Retrieved from https://www.cdc.gov/media/releases/2017/p0718-diabetes-report.html

Chen, A., & Ashburn, M. A. (2015). Cardiac effects of opioid therapy. *Pain Medicine, 16 Suppl 1*, S27-31. doi:10.1111/pme.12915

Colberg, S. R., Sigal, R. J., Fernhall, B., Regensteiner, J. G., Blissmer, B. J., Rubin, R. R., . . . Braun, B. (2010). Exercise and type 2 diabetes: The American College of Sports Medicine and the American Diabetes Association: Joint position statement. *Diabetes Care, 33*(12), e147-167. doi:10.2337/dc10-9990

Colberg, S. R., Sigal, R. J., Yardley, J. E., Riddell, M. C., Dunstan, D. W., Dempsey, P. C., . . . Tate, D. F. (2016). Physical activity/exercise and diabetes: A position statement of the American Diabetes Association. *Diabetes Care, 39*(11), 2065-2079. doi:10.2337/dc16-1728

Convertino, V. A., Armstrong, L. E., Coyle, E. F., Mack, G. W., Sawka, M. N., Senay, L. C., Jr., & Sherman, W. M. (1996). American College of Sports Medicine position stand. Exercise and fluid replacement. *Medicine & Science in Sports & Exercise, 28*(1), i-vii.

Geneen, L. J., Moore, R. A., Clarke, C., Martin, D., Colvin, L. A., & Smith, B. H. (2017). Physical activity and exercise for chronic pain in adults: An overview of Cochrane Reviews. *Cochrane Database of Systematic Reviews, 4*, Cd011279. doi:10.1002/14651858.CD011279.pub3

Gillinov, S., Etiwy, M., Wang, R., Blackburn, G., Phelan, D., Gillinov, A. M., . . . Desai, M. Y. (2017). Variable accuracy of wearable heart rate monitors during aerobic exercise. *Medicine & Science in Sports & Exercise, 49*(8), 1697-1703. doi:10.1249/mss.0000000000001284

Gordon, N. F., & Duncan, J. J. (1991). Effect of beta-blockers on exercise physiology: Implications for exercise training. *Medicine & Science in Sports & Exercise, 23*(6), 668-676.

Reference

Kindermann, W. (1987). Calcium antagonists and exercise performance. *Sports Medicine,* *4*(3), 177-193. doi:10.2165/00007256-198704030-00003

Laukkanen, R. M., & Virtanen, P. K. (1998). Heart rate monitors: state of the art. *Journal of Sports Sciences, 16 Suppl*, S3-7. doi:10.1080/026404198366920

Lopez-Saca, J. M., & Centeno, C. (2014). Opioids prescription for symptoms relief and the impact on respiratory function: updated evidence. *Current Opinion in Supportive and Palliative Care, 8*(4), 383-390. doi:10.1097/spc.0000000000000098

Lundberg, T. R., & Howatson, G. (2018). Analgesic and anti-inflammatory drugs in sports: Implications for exercise performance and training adaptations. *Scandinavian Journal of Medicine & Science in Sports, 28*(11), 2252-2262. doi:10.1111/sms.13275

McGowan, C. J., Pyne, D. B., Thompson, K. G., & Rattray, B. (2015). Warm-up strategies for sport and exercise: Mechanisms and applications. *Sports Medicine, 45*(11), 1523-1546. doi:10.1007/s40279-015-0376-x

Medicine, A. C. o. S. (2018). *ACSM's Guidelines for Exercise Testing and Prescription 10th Edition*. Philadelphia, PA: Wolters Kluwer.

Meeusen, R., Piacentini, M. F., Van Den Eynde, S., Magnus, L., & De Meirleir, K. (2001). Exercise performance is not influenced by a 5-HT reuptake inhibitor. *International Journal in Sports Medicine, 22*(5), 329-336. doi:10.1055/s-2001-15648

Parise, G., Bosman, M. J., Boecker, D. R., Barry, M. J., & Tarnopolsky, M. A. (2001). Selective serotonin reuptake inhibitors: Their effect on high-intensity exercise performance. *Archives of Physical Medicine and Rehabilitation, 82*(7), 867-871. doi:10.1053/apmr.2001.23275

Pescatello, L. S., Franklin, B. A., Fagard, R., Farquhar, W. B., Kelley, G. A., & Ray, C. A. (2004). American College of Sports Medicine position stand. Exercise and hypertension. *Medicine & Science in Sports & Exercise, 36*(3), 533-553.

Pescatello, L. S., MacDonald, H. V., Lamberti, L., & Johnson, B. T. (2015). Exercise for hypertension: A prescription update integrating existing recommendations with emerging research. *Current Hypertension Reports, 17*(11), 87. doi:10.1007/s11906-015-0600-y

Reed, J. L., & Pipe, A. L. (2014). The talk test: A useful tool for prescribing and monitoring exercise intensity. *Current Opinion in Cardiology, 29*(5), 475-480. doi:10.1097/hco.0000000000000097

Rizzo, L., & Thompson, M. W. (2018). Cardiovascular adjustments to heat stress during prolonged exercise. *Journal of Sports Medicine and Physical Fitness, 58*(5), 727-743. doi:10.23736/s0022-4707.17.06831-1

Schuch, F. B., Vancampfort, D., Richards, J., Rosenbaum, S., Ward, P. B., & Stubbs, B. (2016). Exercise as a treatment for depression: A meta-analysis adjusting for publication bias. *Journal of Psychiatric Research, 77*, 42-51. doi:10.1016/j.jpsychires.2016.02.023

Van Hooren, B., & Peake, J. M. (2018). Do we need a cool-down after exercise? A narrative review of the psychophysiological effects and the effects on performance, injuries and the long-term adaptive response. *Sports Medicine, 48*(7), 1575-1595. doi:10.1007/s40279-018-0916-2

Wang, R., Blackburn, G., Desai, M., Phelan, D., Gillinov, L., Houghtaling, P., & Gillinov, M. (2017). Accuracy of wrist-worn heart rate monitors. *JAMA Cardiology, 2*(1), 104-106. doi:10.1001/jamacardio.2016.3340

Wilmore, J., & Costill, D. (2005). *Physiology of Sport and Exercise* (3rd ed.). Champaign, IL: Human Kinetics.

Chapter 9

Barreto Pde, S., Demougeot, L., Pillard, F., Lapeyre-Mestre, M., & Rolland, Y. (2015). Exercise training for managing behavioral and psychological symptoms in people with dementia: A systematic review and meta-analysis. *Ageing Research Reviews, 24*(Pt B), 274-285. doi:10.1016/j.arr.2015.09.001

Black, W., & Almeida, O. P. (2004). A systematic review of the association between the behavioral and psychological symptoms of dementia and burden of care. *International Psychogeriatrics, 16*(3), 295-315.

Carson, S., McDonagh, M. S., & Peterson, K. (2006). A systematic review of the efficacy and safety of atypical antipsychotics in patients with psychological and behavioral symptoms of dementia. *Journal of the American Geriatrics Society, 54*(2), 354-361. doi:10.1111/j.1532-5415.2005.00566.x

Daiello, L. A., Beier, M. T., Hoffmann, V. P., & Kennedy, J. S. (2003). Pharmacotherapy of behavioral and psychological symptoms of dementia: A review of atypical antipsychotics. *Consult Pharm, 18*(2), 138-152, 155-137.

Fleiner, T., Leucht, S., Forstl, H., Zijlstra, W., & Haussermann, P. (2017). Effects of short-term exercise interventions on behavioral and psychological symptoms in patients with dementia: A systematic review. *Journal of Alzheimer's Disease, 55*(4), 1583-1594. doi:10.3233/JAD-160683

Gaugler, J. E., Yu, F., Davila, H. W., & Shippee, T. (2014). Alzheimer's disease and nursing homes. *Health affairs, 33*(4), 650-657. doi:10.1377/hlthaff.2013.1268

Gaugler, J. E., Yu, F., Krichbaum, K., & Wyman, J. F. (2009). Predictors of nursing home admission for persons with dementia. *Medical Care, 47*(2), 191-198.

Henry, G., Williamson, D., & Tampi, R. R. (2011). Efficacy and tolerability of antidepressants in the treatment of behavioral and psychological symptoms of dementia, a literature review of evidence. *American Journal of Alzheimer's Disease and Other Dementias, 26*(3), 169-183. doi:10.1177/1533317511402051

Kolanowski, A., Boltz, M., Galik, E., Gitlin, L. N., Kales, H. C., Resnick, B., . . . Scerpella, D. (2017). Determinants of behavioral and psychological symptoms of dementia: A scoping review of the evidence. *Nursing Outlook, 65*(5), 515-529. doi:10.1016/j.outlook.2017.06.006

Konovalov, S., Muralee, S., & Tampi, R. R. (2008). Anticonvulsants for the treatment of behavioral and psychological symptoms of dementia: A literature review. *International Psychogeriatrics, 20*(2), 293-308. doi:10.1017/S1041610207006540

Laks, J., & Engelhardt, E. (2008). Behavioral and psychological symptoms in dementia is not a unitary concept: A critical review with emphasis on Alzheimer's disease. *Dementia & Neuropsychologia, 2*(4), 272-277. doi:10.1590/S1980-57642009DN20400007

Ornstein, K., & Gaugler, J. E. (2012). The problem with "problem behaviors": A systematic review of the association between individual patient behavioral and psychological symptoms and caregiver depression and burden within the dementia patient-caregiver dyad. *International Psychogeriatrics, 24*(10), 1536-1552. doi:10.1017/S1041610212000737

Preuss, U. W., Wong, J. W., & Koller, G. (2016). Treatment of behavioral and psychological symptoms of dementia: A systematic review. *Psychiatria Polska, 50*(4), 679-715. doi:10.12740/PP/64477

Rodda, J., Morgan, S., & Walker, Z. (2009). Are cholinesterase inhibitors effective in the management of the behavioral and psychological symptoms of dementia in Alzheimer's disease? A systematic review of randomized, placebo-controlled trials of donepezil, rivastigmine and galantamine. *International Psychogeriatrics,* 21(5), 813-824. doi:10.1017/S1041610209990354

Tampi, R. R., Hassell, C., Joshi, P., & Tampi, D. J. (2017). Analgesics in the management of behavioral and psychological symptoms of dementia: A perspective review. *Drugs Context, 6,* 212508. doi:10.7573/dic.212508

Tampi, R. R., & Tampi, D. J. (2014). Efficacy and tolerability of benzodiazepines for the treatment of behavioral and psychological symptoms of dementia: A systematic review of randomized controlled trials. *American Journal of Alzheimer's Disease and Other Dementias,* 29(7), 565-574. doi:10.1177/1533317514524813

Testad, I., Corbett, A., Aarsland, D., Lexow, K. O., Fossey, J., Woods, B., & Ballard, C. (2014). The value of personalized psychosocial interventions to address behavioral and psychological symptoms in people with dementia living in care home settings: A systematic review. *International Psychogeriatrics,* 26(7), 1083-1098. doi:10.1017/S1041610214000131

Ueda, T., Suzukamo, Y., Sato, M., & Izumi, S. (2013). Effects of music therapy on behavioral and psychological symptoms of dementia: A systematic review and meta-analysis. *Ageing Research Reviews,* 12(2), 628-641. doi:10.1016/j.arr.2013.02.003

Yeh, Y. C., & Ouyang, W. C. (2012). Mood stabilizers for the treatment of behavioral and psychological symptoms of dementia: an update review. *Kaohsiung Journal of Medical Sciences, 28*(4), 185-193. doi:10.1016/j.kjms.2011.10.025

Chapter 10

Birkenhager-Gillesse, E. G., Kollen, B. J., Achterberg, W. P., Boersma, F., Jongman, L., & Zuidema, S. U. (2018). Effects of psychosocial interventions for behavioral and psychological symptoms in dementia on the prescription of psychotropic drugs: A systematic review and meta-analyses. *Journal of the American Medical Directions Association, 19*(3), 276 e271-276 e279. doi:10.1016/j.jamda.2017.12.100

Cohen-Mansfield, J. (2001). Nonpharmacologic interventions for inappropriate behaviors in dementia: A review, summary, and critique. *American Journal of the Geriatric Psychiatry, 9*(4), 361-381.

de Oliveira, A. M., Radanovic, M., de Mello, P. C., Buchain, P. C., Vizzotto, A. D., Celestino, D. L., . . . Forlenza, O. V. (2015). Nonpharmacological interventions to reduce behavioral and psychological symptoms of dementia: A systematic review. *BioMed Research International, 2015*, 218980. doi:10.1155/2015/218980

Dorey, J. M., Beauchet, O., Thomas Anterion, C., Rouch, I., Krolak-Salmon, P., Gaucher, J., . . . Akiskal, H. S. (2008). Behavioral and psychological symptoms of dementia and bipolar spectrum disorders: Review of the evidence of a relationship and treatment implications. *CNS Spectrums, 13*(9), 796-803.

Jin, B., & Liu, H. (2019). Comparative efficacy and safety of therapy for the behavioral and psychological symptoms of dementia: A systemic review and Bayesian network meta-analysis. *Journal of Neurology*. doi:10.1007/s00415-019-09200-8

Reference

Matsuda, Y., Kishi, T., Shibayama, H., & Iwata, N. (2013). Yokukansan in the treatment of behavioral and psychological symptoms of dementia: A systematic review and meta-analysis of randomized controlled trials. *Human Psychopharmacology, 28*(1), 80-86. doi:10.1002/hup.2286

Ornstein, K., & Gaugler, J. E. (2012). The problem with "problem behaviors": A systematic review of the association between individual patient behavioral and psychological symptoms and caregiver depression and burden within the dementia patient-caregiver dyad. *International Psychogeriatrics, 24*(10), 1536-1552. doi:10.1017/S1041610212000737

Preuss, U. W., Wong, J. W., & Koller, G. (2016). Treatment of behavioral and psychological symptoms of dementia: A systematic review. *Psychiatriatria Polska, 50*(4), 679-715. doi:10.12740/PP/64477

Tsoi, K. K. F., Chan, J. Y. C., Ng, Y. M., Lee, M. M. Y.,

Kwok, T. C. Y., & Wong, S. Y. S. (2018). Receptive music therapy is more effective than interactive music therapy to relieve behavioral and psychological symptoms of dementia: A systematic review and meta-analysis. *Journal of the American Medical Directors Association, 19*(7), 568-576 e563. doi:10.1016/j.jamda.2017.12.009

Chapter 11

Derouesne, C., Lagha-Pierucci, S., Thibault, S., Baudouin-Madec, V., Lacomblez, L. (2000). Apraxic disturbances in patients with mild to moderate Alzheimer's disease. *Neuropsychologia*, 38(13),1760-1769.

Femminella, G.D., Rengo, G., Komici, K. (2014) Autonomic dysfunction in Alzheimer's disease: Tools for assessment and review of the literature. *Journal of Alzheimer's Disease*, 42(2), 369-377.

Goldman, W.P., Baty, J.D., Buckles, V.D., Sahrmann, S., Morris, J.C. (1999) Motor dysfunction in mildly demented AD individuals without extrapyramidal signs. *Neurology*, 53(5), 956-962.

McCorry, L.K. (2007) Physiology of the autonomic nervous system. *The American Journal of Pharmaceutical Education*, 71(4), 78.

Morris, J.K., Honea, R.A., Vidoni, E.D., Swerdlow, R.H., Burns, J.M. (2014) Is Alzheimer's disease a systemic disease? *Biochimica et Biophysica Acta*, 1842(9),1340-1349.

Yu, F., Bil, K. (2010) Correlating heart rate and perceived exertion during aerobic exercise in Alzheimer's disease. *Nursing and Health Sciences*, 12(3), 375-380.

Yu, F., Demorest, S.L., Vock, D.M. (2015) Testing a modified perceived exertion scale for *Alzheimer's disease*. *PsyCh Journal*, 4(1), 38-46.

Glossary

ABC-MESSS Tool: a tool used for BPSD prevention and treatment. ABC-MESSS is the acronym of AD education; Behavioral modification; Cognition- and emotion-oriented interventions; Medical and nursing interventions; Environmental design; Social interaction; Structured activities; and Sensory enhancement or relaxation.

Abstraction: the classification of higher concepts based on the general attributes of concrete concepts.

AD continuum: AD abnormal processes in the brain are continuous with no fixed events the beginning and end of an AD phase.

AD phases: the clinical course of AD is divided into three phases as preclinical AD, MCI due to AD, and Alzheimer's dementia.

Aerobic exercise: continuous, rhythmic movements of body parts (e.g., legs, arms) that provide cardiorespiratory conditioning. Aerobic exercise is also known as cardiorespiratory or endurance exercise.

Aerobic fitness or cardiorespiratory fitness: the ability of the body's cardiovascular and respiratory systems to supply oxygen to working skeletal muscles for energy production during sustained physical activity.

Aggression: a hostile, forceful behavior or disposition directed at a person or the environment.

Agitation: a broad category of symptoms that includes restlessness, pacing, arguing, disruptive vocalizations, and resistance to care (e.g., rejecting other people's assistance in activities such as bathing, dressing, and grooming).

Alzheimer's dementia: dementia that is caused by AD abnormal brain changes and is the most common type of dementia.

Alzheimer's disease: abnormal changes in the brain which are marked by amyloid plaques and neurofibrillary tangles as well as other changes.

Amyloid plaques: clusters of Aβ which deposit diffusely in the brain and attract each other to form interlaced fibrils and fibrils then stick to each other to form β sheets which in turn fold into each other to form amyloid plaque.

Amyloid-beta or Aβ: amyloid proteins that are increasingly produced in AD and are 38 to 43 amino-acid long.

Anxiety: excessive fear or worry and other symptoms that make it hard to carry out daily activities and responsibilities.

Apathy: a cluster of motivational deficits expressed by a lack of feeling, emotion, interest, or concern.

Apolipoprotein E (*APOE*) gene allele 4 (ε4): the presence of one form (ε4) of the APOE gene which increases the risk for AD.

Approach AD S.A.F.E.ly™ effective communication: assessing the communication ability of people with Alzheimer's dementia and adapting communication styles to meet them where they are.

Approach AD S.A.F.E.ly™ protocol: our recently named brand which originated from pre-exercise health screening and includes all aspects of safely engaging people with Alzheimer's dementia in exercise.

Glossary

AT(N) system: a system to classify AD biomarkers into three categories: A (amyloid), T (tau), and N (neurodegeneration or neuronal injury).

Attention: the ability to focus (sustained attention), selectively concentrate on some aspects of the environment while ignoring others (selective attention), and focus on multiple tasks simultaneously (divided attention).

Awareness: insight of people with Alzheimer's dementia about their dementia and its severity and impact on their ability to carry out daily activities.

Balance or neuromuscular exercise: exercise that challenges balance and proprioception or awareness of one's position and movement.

Balance: the ability to stay upright or in control of body movement and can be classified as static and dynamic balance.

Behavioral and psychological symptoms of dementia or BPSD: symptoms that are common in people with dementia, including depression, anxiety, psychosis (hallucinations and delusions), apathy, loss of normal inhibitions, sleep disturbances, agitation, and aggression.

BEIC Tool: a tool to work with family caregivers. BEIC, pronounced "bake," stands for Befriend, Empathize, Identify, and Communicate.

Biomarker: an indicator of normal biological processes, pathogenic processes, or responses to treatments.

Body composition: the percentages of fat and fat-free mass (e.g., water, muscle, and bone). Both body fat and fat-free mass predict the likelihood of dying from any causes.

Brain reserve: the brain's ability to tolerate injury by showing no or few symptoms of cognitive impairment.

Cardiovascular conditions: heart- and blood vessel-related conditions.

Cerebrospinal fluid or CSF: a clear and colorless fluid circulating the hollow cavities in the brain called the ventricles. The CSF contains mainly proteins and electrolytes, with few cells. Changes in the CSF contents can indicate changes in the brain.

Cognition: the mental processes of knowing and can be divided into different domains.

Cognitive flexibility: the ability to adapt to a change by getting the integrated information ready to make the next move.

Cognitive reserve: the brain's ability to compensate for injury using alternative brain networks or cognitive strategies.

Cool-down: performing aerobic exercise at a slower than normal pace for five to 10 minutes after the stimulus phase.

Cortex: the surface of the cerebrum.

Cortical thickness: a measure of how thick the gray matter is.

Dementia: a clinical syndrome of cognitive impairment, functional decline, and behavioral psychological symptoms of dementia. It is an umbrella term with many different types or causes.

Depression: depressed mood and markedly diminished interest or pleasure in all, or almost all, activities.

Diagnostic criteria: the criteria used by health care providers to make a diagnosis of a medical condition.

Disinhibition: undue familiarity and impulsive comments and actions shown by a lack of restraint, such as disregard of social norms and impulsivity.

Episodic memory: the conscious recollection of experienced events at certain times and places as well as their social and physical contexts.

Executive function: a higher-order cognitive construct and involves a set of skills that organize and regulate goal-directed behaviors and effective use of large amounts of information. It includes working memory, cognitive flexibility, and inhibitory control.

Glossary

Exercise provider: anyone who plans and supervises exercise sessions for other people, including personal trainers, aerobics instructors, physical therapists, occupational therapists, recreational therapists, activity directors, exercise physiologists, nurses, and physicians.

Exercise specialists: exercise providers trained in engaging people with Alzheimer's dementia in exercise.

Exercise: a type of physical activity that is "planned, structured, and repetitive bodily movement done to improve or maintain one or more components of physical fitness" per ACSM, according to the American College of Sports Medicine.

Exertion signs and symptoms: subjectively reported symptoms or objectively observed signs indicating exercise exertion levels.

Fall: suddenly come to a lower level without intention to get there.

Family caregiver: is a family member, friend, or other helper who takes care of another person.

Fear of falling: being afraid of going to fall.

FITT-VP: the acronym representing Frequency (how often), Intensity (how hard), Time (duration, or how long), Type (mode or what kind), Volume (how much or amount—a combination of Frequency, Intensity, and Time), and Progression (advancement).

Flexibility exercise or stretching: exercise that extends a body part.

Flexibility: the ability to move a joint through a complete range of motion.

Frontal lobes: the front section of the brain behind the forehead and are associated with executive function, personality, emotions, parts of speech (speaking and writing), body movement, intelligence, concentration, and self-awareness.

Functional decline: decrease from a previously higher level of functioning in advanced, instrumental, and basic activities of daily living.

Genetic risk: the presence of a certain gene or mutation in a gene that increases the risk of disease.

Gray matter: neural tissues that contain nerve-cell bodies and fibers and gives cortex the pinkish-gray coloring.

HAPI Tool: a tool to get to know people with Alzheimer's dementia. HAPI is pronounced as "happy" and stands for: Have the right attitude; Ask the family caregiver, Pick out a routine that works for everyone; and Initiate on day one.

Heart rate reserve: the difference in peak heart rate during aerobic fitness testing and resting heart rate.

Heart rate: the number of heartbeats per minute.

High-intensity interval training or HIIT: a few minutes of high-intensity exercise alternating with several minutes of low-intensity exercise.

Hippocampus: the seahorse-like brain structure located within the temporal lobes where memory is formed.

Hyperphosphorylated tau: the overload of extra phosphate to normal tau.

Implicit memory: the memory that can be recalled automatically without conscious effort and be expressed by means other than words.

Inflamm-aging: a chronic, low-grade systemic inflammation linked with normal aging.

Inhibitory control: the ability to suppress the information and behaviors that are not pertinent to the task at hand.

Insulin resistance: the inhibition of the brain cells' ability to use insulin effectively and might result from decreased insulin receptors.

Intelligence: the patterns of cognitive change over time.

Judgment and problem solving: the ability to make decisions, come to sensible conclusions, and solve problems.

Glossary

Language: the ability to produce spontaneous speech, comprehend and repeat language, name objects, read, and write.

Leaky guts: increased permeability and/or decreased barrier function of the intestines.

Lobe: a section of the cortex. The cortex is divided into four lobes by the distinct hills called gyri and valleys named sulci: the frontal, parietal, temporal, and occipital lobes.

Magnetic resonance imaging or MRI: a noninvasive imaging method of the brain to identify structural (structural MRI) and functional changes (functional MRI) in the brain.

Memory: the ability to encode, store, and retrieve information.

Microbiome: the trillions of microorganisms such as bacteria, fungi, and other microbes that exist inside the intestines and on the skin.

Mild cognitive impairment due to AD: the period between preclinical AD and the full development of Alzheimer's dementia. It is a clinical diagnosis.

Mitochondria cascade hypothesis: mitochondria dysfunction occurs with aging and is influenced by a person's genetics and environment. Once mitochondrial dysfunction reaches a critical tipping point, AD hallmark brain changes, neurodegeneration, and oxidative stress ensue.

Modifiable risk factors: risk factors are changeable so actions can be taken to reduce the risk.

Muscle strength: a measure of muscle fitness and is defined as the maximum amount of force muscle can exert against some form of resistance at a single time.

Neurodegeneration: synaptic dysfunction and loss as well as neuronal injury and death.

Neurofibrillary tangles: clusters of hyperphosphorylated tau proteins within the neurons in AD.

Neuroinflammation: a vital part of the brain's self-defense system that activates the brain's immune cells to eliminate pathogens (such as bacteria and viruses) and cellular debris.

Neurotransmitters: the chemical messengers released to the synapses when neural impulses arrive.

Non-exercise or leisure-time physical activity: activities embedded in daily life.

Occipital lobes: the back of the head and regulate visual processing of color, light, and movement.

Oxidative stress: physiological stress caused by damage from free radicals that are not adequately removed by antioxidants.

Parietal lobes: the top middle section of the brain above the ears and affect speech (language interpretation and words), spatial and visual perceptions, and interpretation of visual and auditory signals as well as senses of touch, pain, and temperature.

Person-centered care: individualized and coordinated care given within a person's context, which supports personhood with compassion and respect for dignity.

Physical activity: a bodily movement that is produced by the contraction of skeletal muscles and that substantially increases energy expenditure, according to the American College of Sports Medicine.

Physical fitness: an umbrella term with five components: aerobic fitness, muscular fitness, body composition, balance, and flexibility.

Positron emission tomography or PET: a minimally invasive imaging method of the brain which requires the injection of a radioactive tracer to the peripheral blood that binds to amyloid (amyloid PET), tau (tau PET), or glucose (fluorodeoxyglucose or FDG PET) in the brain.

Glossary

Preclinical AD: refers to the years or decades in which AD brain changes begin to develop and build-up, but it is not a clinical diagnosis.

Processing speed: the speed of performing cognitive activities and motor responses.

Protective factors: factors that protect against the development of a disease and/or can slow down the progression of a disease.

Psychosis: "gross impairment in reality testing" or "loss of ego boundaries" that interferes with a person's ability to carry out daily activities. Psychosis includes delusion and hallucination.

RECUSS Tool: a tool to motivate people with Alzheimer's dementia to exercise. RECUSS, pronounced "recess," stands for Rely on rapport with your client, Establish an enjoyable environment, Capitalize on social support, Understand your influence, Sing praises for effort, and Support family caregivers.

Risk factors: factors that predict the onset and progression of a disease and provide targets for developing treatments.

S.A.F.E. Tool: a tool to conduct pre-exercise health screening. S.A.F.E. stands for 1) Screen your conditions, 2) Assess exercise readiness, 3) Follow medical evaluation, if needed; and 4) Evaluate aerobic fitness.

Sedentary behavior: too much sitting.

Sleep disturbances: sleep-related changes such as poor sleep quality and long durations of sleep (> eight hours).

SLO-BUTS Tool: a tool to communicate with people with Alzheimer's dementia. SLO-BUTS, pronounced as "slow buzz," is the acronym of Speak in short sentences; Limit choices; Orient people with Alzheimer's dementia; Break down tasks; Use concrete words; Talk with eye contact and appropriate body language; and Slash distractions.

Stages of Alzheimer's dementia: the clinical course of Alzheimer's dementia is divided into mild (early), moderate (middle), and severe (late) stages based on the severity of symptoms and the need for assistance.

Stimulus phase: the target dose of the aerobic exercise session is performed after the warm-up.

Strength exercise: exercise that causes the muscles to contract against external resistance to increase strength, muscle mass, and muscle endurance. Strength exercise is also called muscle building, weight lifting, and resistance exercise.

Subcortical: below the cortex.

Subjective cognitive decline or SCD: cognitive symptoms are noticeable to the person affected.

Synapse: the point where nervous impulse passes from one neuron to another.

Syndrome: a group of symptoms that occur together consistently.

Talk test: the ability to talk a sentence while breathing patterns are observed.

Target exercise dose: 150 minutes of moderate-intensity aerobic exercise a week for promoting brain health, preventing AD, and treating AD symptoms.

Temporal lobes: the bottom section of the brain around the ears and control memory, understanding of language, hearing, sequencing, and organization.

Tip-of-the-tongue: the experience of word-finding problems although the word is known.

Transgenic animal models: animals with genes taken from one organism and transferred into the genetic makeup of another.

Traumatic brain injury: a sudden trauma to the brain through an abrupt and forceful collision with an object, a whiplash-like incident, or an object that pierces the skull and damages the brain tissue.

Glossary

Vascular dysfunction: the presence of cerebral small vessel disease, cardiovascular conditions and risk factors, or vascular dementia.

Verbal fluency: information retrieval from memory.

Visuospatial function: the ability to perceive, comprehend, and interpret visual and spatial information in different dimensions.

Warm-up: starting exercise at a low intensity and then gradually increasing the intensity until reaching the target exercise dose.

Working memory: the memory that temporarily stores short-term memory and calls up information from other areas of the brain to integrate all information together and with past experience.

Index

Index

About the Authors

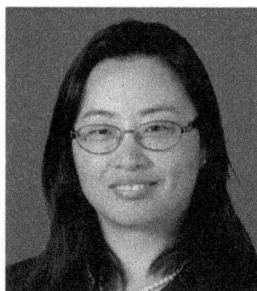

Fang Yu, PhD, RN, FGSA, FAAN, is a Professor and Chair of the Adult and Gerontological Health Cooperative Unit and holds the Long-Term Care Professorship at the University of Minnesota School of Nursing. She leads exercise research in Alzheimer's disease (AD) with millions in funding.

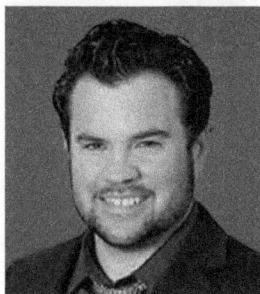

Dereck L. Salisbury, PhD, is an Assistant Professor and Director of the Laboratory of Clinical Physiology at the University of Minnesota School of Nursing. As a clinical exercise physiologist, he focuses on the therapeutic effects of exercise in peripheral artery disease and AD.

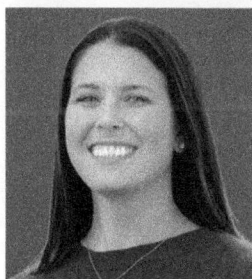

Kaitlin E. Kelly, MSE, ATC, is the Director of Marketing & Life Enrichment at Parks' Place. She became passionate about people with Alzheimer's dementia when working on Yu's FIT-AD™ Trial.